D0120004

# Second Printing

# NOT ALONE
# WITH CANCER

## A Guide for Those Who Care
## What to Expect; What to Do

## RUTH D. ABRAMS, M.S.

*With Forewords by*

**Robert S. Weiss, Ph.D.**
*Associate Professor of Sociology*
*Harvard Medical School*

**John H. Knowles, M.D.**
*President*
*The Rockefeller Foundation*

This volume is intended as a practical and sympathetic guide for all those who have long felt bewildered and frustrated in their attempts to cope with the problems that accompany cancer. Those who are involved with the cancer patient experience heightened and intensified pressures as they labor to care for the patient.

NOT ALONE WITH CANCER offers suggestions for management which are specific for each care-giver, with the goal of maintaining mutually stable and satisfying relationships as well as securing the patient's comfort. The book explains what to expect and what to do at each of the three recognized stages of the disease. The proposed formula is presented in such a way as to be clearly defined, factual and practical.

CHARLES C THOMAS • PUBLISHER • SPRINGFIELD • ILLINOIS

# NOT ALONE
# WITH CANCER

*Supported in part*
*by*

A Private Foundation
Cambridge, Massachusetts

*and*

The American Cancer Society, Inc.
New York, New York

*Second Printing*

# NOT ALONE
# WITH CANCER

## A Guide for Those Who Care
## What to Expect; What to Do

*By*

RUTH D. ABRAMS, M.S.

*With Forewords by*

Robert S. Weiss, Ph.D.
*Associate Professor of Sociology*
*Harvard Medical School*

*and*

John H. Knowles, M.D.
*President*
*The Rockefeller Foundation*

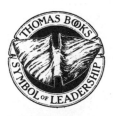

CHARLES C THOMAS • PUBLISHER
*Springfield • Illinois • USA*

1974

*Published and Distributed Throughout the World by*

CHARLES C THOMAS • PUBLISHER

Bannerstone House

301-327 East Lawrence Avenue, Springfield, Illinois, U.S.A.

© *1974 by* CHARLES C THOMAS    PUBLISHER

ISBN 0-398-02973-3

Library of Congress Catalog Card Number: 73-13834

First Printing, 1974
Second Printing, 1976

*Printed in the United States of America*
*R-1*

**Library of Congress Cataloging in Publication Data**

Abrams, Ruth D
    Not alone with cancer.

    Bibliography: p.
    1. Cancer. 2. Cancer—Psychological aspects.
I. Title. [DNLM: 1. Neoplasma—Therapy—Popular
works. 2. Psychotherapy—Popular works. QZ201
A161n 1974]
RC263.A27   1974    616.9'94'0019    73-13834
ISBN 0-398-02973-3

*This book is dedicated to my husband*
**ARCHIE ADAM ABRAMS, M.D.**

# FOREWORD

Henry James wrote a story in which the hero was finally forced to recognize that nothing, absolutely nothing, was going to happen to him. I think James may have intended that the hero exemplify the tragedy of the carefully conducted life, but if so, his story is misleading. For no matter how carefully a man may conduct his life, he cannot escape change, disruption and loss. And at the end of his life, he must deal with that ultimate loss, the loss of himself.

Few of us are truly prepared for the unavoidable crises of living. We see no point in contaminating our present comfort with dark thoughts of fragility. Even as we recognize the vulnerability of our lives to disruption, we banish serious thought about it from our minds. Engaged couples nowadays joke about divorce, but few of them agree in advance how they will divide their property should divorce actually occur. Middle-aged men accept yearly physicals to lessen the likelihood of their early demise, but having done so and having paid their life insurance, they determinedly redirect their attention.

Because we want to protect our confidence in the present, we deny the validity of our own past experience. We dissociate our present normal self from the way we were in a past time of crisis. We say about a time when we were desperately upset over a lost love or a failure at work, that we were not ourselves then, as though that had been a different person who lived in our stead. In consequence we are dismayed when we respond to a new crisis as we responded to an earlier one.

This is not to say we never learn from our own experience; sometimes we learn too well. Particularly if we have been badly hurt and cannot understand why — if, for example, we suddenly, inexplicably, were rejected by someone we cared for — we may become phobic to a situation in which this might happen again.

But a strategy of avoidance impoverishes our lives without, in the end, truly saving us from stress.

Dissociation of our own past experience is bad enough in leaving us unprepared for new crisis. But we do not simply avoid learning from our own experience; we also avoid learning from that of others. Of course we want to hear about a friend's operation, but not in detail. And we generally do not at all want to know what it feels like to fail at work or in love. A friend who threatens to tell us these things actively embarrasses us. And so we prepare ourselves to be confounded by failure or loss when they happen to us.

Because we learn little from our own past or from the present lives of others, each of us, when within a crisis, experiences it as though it had never happened before. Our very ignorance of what is happening becomes one of our difficulties. We do not know what to expect of ourselves or others. We cannot judge the end point of the trajectory along which we find ourselves moving. To give an example: New widows and widowers often are for a time overwhelmed by feelings of grief to the point of near inability to function. They suppose that it must soon become obvious to others as well as to themselves that they have lost control, and they fear that institutionalization may yet await them. This is by no means an unusual early reaction to devastating loss and is entirely compatible with eventual recovery. But because each bereaved individual experiences it without awareness of its normality, each is liable to add fear of personal disintegration to grief over loss.

Failure to attend to others when they were in crisis enables us to retain highly idealized models of how crisis should properly be responded to. We hold that divorce should be managed sensibly, without rancor; that the grief of bereavement after a reasonable period should be put aside; that dying should be talked about by the terminally ill openly and with serenity. No one can do any of these things. But because we have not learned this, we are critical of our kin and friends when their response to crisis falls short of our ideal, and we add self-condemnation to our other woes when we, in turn, fall short.

It is extraordinarily helpful for those in crisis to have some sense of what may happen next. Whether they can influence events or not, if they are unable to anticipate, they must constantly be tense, always liable to mistake the trivial for the potentially serious.

Mrs. Abrams has written a volume that fills a desperate need. With both candor and compassion she describes to those who suffer from cancer, and to those others who minister to them, comfort them and suffer with them, the social and emotional implications of cancer.

Mrs. Abrams begins by alerting us to the crucial distinction between the cancer that is localized and constitutes simply a problem to be dealt with before the patient gets on with his life and the cancer that is widespread and signals the imminent end of the road. When cancer is localized, it can be dealt with as might be any other threat. The individual can seek help from family as well as professionals for vanquishing it. But when cancer is widespread, it is more difficult to seek allies for this losing cause. One values those who can help restrain it, but now one avoids revealing its presence to others, as one would avoid revealing any other unacceptable aspect of the self.

There are other reasons why individuals prefer to be secretive about widespread cancer. To declare oneself moribund would establish one as irrelevant to any future-oriented discussion. The individual who knows his time is limited cannot share that knowledge lest he become a lame duck among the living.

And there is tact. How tactless it would be of the dying to admit their condition! To do so would induce not only sympathy but perhaps also guilt and terror in their audience. Certainly, it would disturb the feelings of well-being of those around. Nor is this an unworthy consideration. None of us can respond without hesitancy to those whose lives have been blighted. And yet, the cancer victims must go on living until they actually die, and the quality of their lives will depend on their maintenance of a sustaining web of affiliations. In a better world it would be possible for them to maintain effective ties without dissimulation. In our world generally it is not.

Mrs. Abrams makes clear how freighted with contradictory feelings becomes not only communication, but the very bonds linking the dying patient to those close to him. The dying patient must depend on his family and friends to be guardians of his memory, on his children to be the only living continuations of his self, yet he can hardly help resenting that these other family members will go on living, while he must die. Perhaps the burden of these mixed feelings plays a role in the withdrawal from the family that Mrs. Abrams speaks of as often occurring toward the end. And yet how important it is, despite whatever difficulties there may be, for the family to give care and love to the dying individual, for them to share as much as they can with him in the last months and weeks. It is important for them, so that they can assure themselves later that they gave all they could, as much as it is for the one who is dying.

Mrs. Abrams points out that another issue may burden the reaction of the cancer patient to himself or to those close to him. She recognizes our near compulsion to find explanations for the major events of our lives in terms of what we did or what was done by others to us. It is only human for the cancer patient to ask whether the cancer is his own fault; it seems especially if the genital organs are involved that patients ask whether they might not have misused them. It is equally human to ask whether the cancer may not be a consequence of an injury inflicted inadvertently by someone close to one. Cancer is an assault, and the knowledge that we have cancer causes us to search for its author. It is difficult to accept that personal disaster may have no personal cause.

There is a value system implicit in Mrs. Abrams' book regarding how one should deal with those who have suffered major reverse, and it may be well to make it explicit. It is a value system in which dignity and the continued capacity to meet obligations to self and others rank higher than "openness" or "good communication." Mrs. Abrams observes that the patient with advanced cancer, for reasons already noted, no longer finds it easy to talk candidly about his condition. Her response is not to recommend insight therapy or family councils, or group discussions that might serve to dilute defenses and encourage talk. She recognizes that the barriers to communication are introduced for good reason. If that is the way the patient handles it best, Mrs. Abrams says, let him be.

Mrs. Abrams adopts the same position in relation to the dying patient's changed view of his physician. It is perhaps only for the dying patient that a physician genuinely approaches the status of God, for within narrow limits the physician can in fact decide the range and quality of the patient's future. The directions and appraisals of the physician naturally come to matter more than those of the family. But this too initiates some withdrawal from the family. Mrs. Abrams advises that the withdrawal be understood and accepted for what it is: not repudiation of the family, but rather acceptance that it is no longer family members who control one's well-being.

Although Mrs. Abrams writes primarily for those directly or indirectly engaged with cancer, she raises issues of fundamental importance for everyone. When she discusses, in passing, the different ways individuals react to learning that their lives are approaching their ends, she makes us wonder what we would do were we to receive that message. Having come this far, we wonder about the way we live our lives now. The development of hospitals and the minimization of mourning ritual have together managed to remove many of the *momento mori* that once were a part of ordinary life, although the funeral home just outside the suburban business district, the cemetery at the city's outskirts and the obituary column in the daily newspaper may nevertheless remind us of mortality. Mrs. Abrams, by spelling out what happens at the end of life, forces us to recognize that time has us, too, in its grip, and that we, too, will have our confrontation with death. What self, with what history, shall we bring to that confrontation? Despite our reluctance, Mrs. Abrams encourages us to prepare ourselves.

ROBERT S. WEISS, Ph.D.
Associate Professor of Sociology
Department of Psychiatry
Harvard Medical School
Boston, Massachusetts

# FOREWORD

I FIRST met Ruth Abrams in the Emergency Ward of the Massachusetts General Hospital in 1953, when we shared the care of a patient with terminal disease of the lungs. It was my best experience in the art and science of medicine. I had always believed deeply that medicine is a social as well as a biological science, and Ruth Abrams showed me what medical social work can do in the total effort to succor the sick. She always worked with such a rare combination of head and heart — knowledge and compassion — that I wished there were a thousand like her. When she told me she had written a book on the best care of the cancer patient, I was delighted to be asked to add this foreword for a good old friend and one who has always exemplified the best in medical social work.

As Ruth Abrams herself says, every patient with cancer — no matter what stage of the disease he or she is in — has the human right to be part of the treatment team, and each member of the caring team must think first of the patient's needs and wishes before considering his or her own. Cancer remains the most feared disease that afflicts humanity. Its incidence continues to increase, and it is the second leading cause of death in the United States. Science and technology have done much to reduce the morbidity and mortality of the disease and to alleviate the attendant suffering. The human skills and the personal elements of caring have not progressed as rapidly, and the team approach to the best care of the cancer patient has only recently received the attention it deserves. Ruth Abrams' book can be read profitably by professionals and lay people alike, for it distills a long experience with the care of cancer patients — an experience which has combined knowledge and kindness in the act of caring for the sick. It is a pleasure to acknowledge her contribution with this fine book and to salute her and the Massachusetts General

xiii

Hospital, where medical social work was first begun at the turn of the century.

John H. Knowles, M.D.
President, The Rockefeller Foundation

# PREFACE

A WISE doctor, the professor of research medicine at the Harvard Medical School, greeted me in the Tumor Clinic of Massachusetts General Hospital twenty-five years ago with the remark, "I have only one word of advice: Make as few mistakes as possible. These you will never forget, but your successes are quickly forgotten."

Those words rang in my ears at 1 pm one Saturday afternoon just as the Gynecological Tumor Clinic was closing. I heard a scream from the examining room. It was not a cry of physical pain but of another kind of anguish. A moment later the chief of the service, one of the leading gynecologists in the country, ran into my office. "You'll have to take over," he cried. "I have just told Mrs. Rossi* that she has cancer and that it has already spread. You know how emotional these Italians are. But she drove me to telling her the truth."

So there I was, a well-trained social worker with all the right credentials, a woman in her thirties, married to a doctor, mother of two children, and yet totally unprepared for this patient. How to comfort her? How even to handle my own mounting anxieties?

I was like the patient in one way. We were both caught in a new experience — and we were alone. Everyone had left the clinic for the day — doctors, medical students, nurses, secretaries. No other social worker was available, and even if there had been one, how could I turn away for help without increasing Mrs. Rossi's fears? She as the patient, and I as the only professional helper in sight, had somehow to manage ourselves and give one another something toward establishing a relationship of mutual trust.

All I had was the bulky medical record indicating that she had

---

*Not her real name.

been at Massachusetts General Hospital for a long time, but she was already in my office before I could scan it.

I started by letting Mrs. Rossi tell her story in her own way. She avoided any reference to what the chief had actually told her and never used the word cancer. However, she did say that no matter what course her illness took she would remain at home and train her girls so that they would be prepared to care for the home and her husband when she was no longer there. She did not mention what she would tell her family on her return home, and I deliberately did not ask her. Rather she focused on her present and past life, emphasizing the good things she had had. Obviously she was much more courageous than I. All I could do was listen with empathy and inform her that there were specific services in the community that might prove helpful now or later. I did emphasize the fact that I would stand by and be available indefinitely whether she came to the hospital regularly, or not at all.

So I learned my first lesson. Listen to the patient, she will tell you how much, how little and with whom she wishes to discuss her fears or anxieties. Above all let her make the choices that she, rather than you, her caregiver, can tolerate. Regardless of the outlook, let her manage the course of her life and herself to the best of her ability.

Another lesson I learned from the case was invaluable. The following week I sought out the doctor who had sent her to me and asked, "Would you tell me what you tell your patients with cancer?" He answered quickly, "With my ward patients I rarely tell them anything, but with my private patients I am apt to give them a good deal of the truth." "Why the difference?" I asked. Again his answer was prompt and assured. "You see I may not have a chance to know the ward patient well enough to tell her what I think she really wants to know and I probably will not see her again. Even if I do, I may forget what I have told her, but I have an opportunity to know my private patients whom I see every day or every other day while they are in the hospital and later in my office. Then I can decide what they really want to know, and they in turn can ask me more if they want to."

I have never forgotten this advice. It made me realize that very few of us know how to help the patient to achieve and maintain an image of himself that both he and his caregivers can tolerate. This principle underlies all that is crucial to the patient's care. The right of the patient with cancer to choose the degree of privacy or communication that he needs and wants has been the focus of my concern throughout my professional life.

Cancer is one of the most dreaded of all diseases; its cause is unknown, its course is unpredictable and its ending is frequently fatal. Furthermore, despite strides made to discover the causes and cures, eradication of the disease still appears to be a long way off.

Yet many people will be surprised to learn that although 329,000 Americans died of cancer in 1970, there are also 1,500,000 Americans alive today who have had cancer and have defeated it. That number is growing every year. These ex-patients are evidence of a hopeful side of cancer that is not so well known. Too many people believe that a diagnosis of cancer means they will die.

Too few people, even if they know that cancer is curable, are aware that the cured cancer patient can return after treatment and a period of convalescence to full-time work and all kinds of other activities. This certainly is not true for the person with heart disease or diabetes — to give two examples. The heart patient usually must curtail some activities and lead a life of moderation. But the cured cancer patient knows that excesses in his life style will not affect cell growth adversely (as far as we know). Believing this, he can more easily be fully rehabilitated and can even forget, eventually, that he had cancer. Perhaps that is why the cured case is not discussed, and the full impact of the curability of cancer has not reached the public.

These are some examples of the progress that is being made against cancer:

Practically all skin cancers are curable.

Cancer of the cervix, when treated early and adequately, frequently is eradicated; this is also true of cancer of the intestines and of other organs.

The life expectancy of persons with chronic forms of leukemia and Hodgkin's disease has been lengthened greatly — sometimes as much as twenty years. During this time the patient lives a normal

*Not Alone With Cancer*

life, with occasional time out for treatment.

Unfortunately, cancer in certain sites — the breast and the lung, for example — continues to show the same rate of mortality as in the past, primarily because they are in silent sites and therefore not readily recognizable until symptoms occur.

With all these reasons for optimism, we cannot seem to take the stigma out of this diagnosis. Why? Is it because cancer is still considered unclean? Do we have guilty thoughts about having the disease?* Why do we need to assign responsibility to ourselves or to someone else for having the disease?† Very commonly a patient will say, "What have I done to deserve it?" A woman will often wonder, "Did I have sexual relations too young? Or too often? Or with too many different partners?" A nurse observed that many women with pelvic lesions can hardly believe that they have these symptoms because "I have always led a clean life" or "I have never abused myself."

The fears and anxieties generated by the disease erect a wall of silence around the patient and those who are involved, frequently presenting barriers to management, adjustment and rehabilitation. Yet those who learn that cancer has invaded their lives are in desperate need of guidance. There are decisions to be made, a new future to be defined, relationships to be re-examined and if necessary mended, specific needs to be met and emotions to be dealt with. All this without preparation or help.

This book has grown out of my nearly twenty-five years of work with the adult patient with cancer and his family, in the capacity of medical and psychiatric social worker, in many clinical and research settings including the Massachusetts General Hospital, the Harvard School of Public Health, the Laboratory of Community Psychiatry, Harvard Medical School and in private practice.

*Not Alone With Cancer* is intended to be a thoughtful and, above all, practical guide to what actually happens when a person gets cancer, with particular emphasis on his psychological reactions and those of his family and the medical team. As the reader

---

*R. D. Abrams, and J. E. Finesinger, Guilt reactions in patients with cancer. *Cancer,* 6:474-482, May 1953.
†H. Shands, J. E. Finesinger, S. Cobb, and R. D. Abrams, Psychological mechanisms in patients with cancer. *Cancer,* 4:1159-1170, 1951.

will see, the patient's manner changes from one of openness to one of withdrawal. There is nothing he can do to improve his condition, and perhaps it is this helplessness that drives him into his shell. I hope this book will show how all involved can understand and cope with the situation in light of what I have found to be the predictability of these reactions. I will make specific suggestions for caring for the patient and his family at each of the three recognized stages of cancer: "localized," "regional involvement" and "advanced."

This book is directed to a varied audience because during this illness the patient and his family have need for supportive services from many different individuals at different times. How often a patient wants from one of his caregivers an immediate response to a psychological problem, or more details about his diagnosis and outlook. It is my earnest wish that a caregiver who wants to be prepared for such a situation will find in this book a measure of hope and help that will be satisfying to himself and to all concerned.

I am not sure where the genesis for this book lies. Perhaps it is in a statement made more than twenty years ago by a dear friend of mine who was in the last stage of acute leukemia. "Long illness is so humiliating," she said. No one answered her remark, including me. Or perhaps it was out of my early experiences as a social worker assigned to the Tumor Clinic of the Massachusetts General Hospital where I worked with patients in various stages of the disease. Gradually, I became aware that the stage of the disease had an emotional impact not only on the patient and his family, but also on the staff. In the early stages they were optimistic, but quite often in the advanced stages, after all efforts to cure or arrest the disease had failed, the medical staff and even the family turned away from the patient. For the sake of continued treatment, the patient repressed his feelings of abandonment and fear. His plight, as well as that of his family, was obvious and tragic. I felt something should be done to alleviate this situation.

In 1966, I published in *The New England Journal of Medicine* an article entitled "The Patient With Cancer — His Changing Pattern of Communication."* In this paper I demonstrated that at

---

*R. D. Abrams, The patient with cancer — his changing pattern of communication. *N Engl J Med, 274*:317-322, February 10, 1966.

each of the recognized stages of the disease the patient changes his pattern of communication and his dependence on the physician, paramedical personnel and family; that recognition of these changes helps add a dimension to effective care. This finding applied to the majority of patients studied regardless of age, sex, marital status, socioeconomic level, sophistication about the disease or site of the lesion.

This article has had a considerable positive response from physicians, surgeons, oncologists, psychiatrists, nurses and chaplains because it describes a formula that is clearly defined, factual and usable. Clinicians and educators suggested that I broaden the scope of my findings to include how and by whom supportive services should be offered to the patient and his family. This book, then, is addressed to professional helpers and family. The patient himself may find the contents helpful and reassuring especially if they coincide with his own experiences and feelings. I do believe that knowing what reactions to expect from cancer patients and their families and what helpful medical and supportive services are available will lessen the burdens imposed by this illness.

It is my hope that this book will live up to the expectations of my colleagues, and that my observations will help break through the wall of silence, uneasiness and despair that has been traditionally, and for too long, a burden to the patient with cancer and those who care for him.

# ACKNOWLEDGMENTS

BEFORE and during the preparation of this book, I was stimulated and encouraged especially by the following members of the helping professions: physicians — Joseph C. Aub, James Feeney, B.J. Kennedy (oncologist) and John H. Knowles; surgeons — Bentley Colcock, the late Joe Vincent Meigs, Howard Ulfelder and Claude E. Welch; psychiatrists — the late Jacob E. Finesinger and Helen H. Tartakoff; nurse — Mira Garland; social worker — the late Ida M. Cannon; sociologist — Robert S. Weiss; attorney — Haskell Cohn; theologian — Rollin J. Fairbanks; and medical editor — Joseph Garland.

Elliot J. Brebner, B.A. and M.S. in engineering and my son-in-law, is responsible for encapsulating my philosophy, goal and purpose with his contribution of the title, NOT ALONE WITH CANCER.

Along the way, I was assisted in the preparation of the manuscript by Diana Potter and Ann Norton. Adelle Robinson was my excellent and loyal typist. To Evelyn Stone and Marlene Hindley I shall be grateful always for their ongoing interest and confidence.

To the American Cancer Society, Inc. and to the private foundation I am indebted for their faith in the plan of the book in terms of providing partial funding.

Thanks are due to the publisher, Charles C Thomas and the help provided by Payne E L Thomas and members of the staff.

Finally, the inspiration for this book was derived in large part from two sources: first, by my patients with cancer and their family members, whether they were courageous or frightened, independent or dependent or even by those who turned away from any or all caregivers; and second, by the many professionals and nonprofessional helpers, who, regardless of their own reactions or involvement cared so deeply that their concern and activity centered not on their own feelings but on those that the patient could tolerate.

# INTRODUCTION

Cancer is usually considered to have three recognized stages: *localized, regional involvement* and *advanced.* *

Stage 1, the *localized* stage, describes the cancer which is contained at the primary site or origin with no evidence of spread to other areas of the body. Medical procedures have much to offer to eradicate this cancer. Prognosis (outlook) is usually good.

Stage 2, the *regional involvement* stage, refers to the lesion (malignant growth) which has spread from the primary site, involving surrounding structures. This spreading is called metastasis. At this stage, the disease may still be controlled by medical procedures, but statistically is not as curable as Stage 1. Prognosis is considered fair to "guarded."

In Stage 3, the *advanced* stage, there is wide metastasis to other parts of the body. Medical procedures are available which may control further growth and extension for a limited or increasingly longer period of time. These procedures usually are applied to provide physical and emotional comfort. The outlook may be considered guarded, but the eventual prognosis is usually poor.

Each of these stages produces a series of crises for the patient, his family and the medical team. In the localized stage, most patients during the treatment period are able to talk freely and repeatedly about their diagnosis with physicians and other persons close to them. With the advent of regional involvement, however, the system of communication becomes disrupted. To defend himself against the knowledge that the initial treatment has not eradicated the disease, the patient's attitudes become cautious, his speech evasive and oblique.

---

*These terms have been designated by the American Cancer Society to take the place of the formerly used words "initial," "advancing" and "terminal."

The patient with advanced cancer faces overwhelming emotional problems: the fear of death itself, the fear of the ordeal of dying and the even more devastating fear of abandonment by his family and caregivers.* His behavioral pattern undergoes a marked change, and overlapping defenses of denial and symptoms of depression dominate his relationships with others. At this time the medical team personnel and more especially the families desperately need to understand that the patient's changed behavior is not a result of something they may or may not have done, but a predictable response to an unbearable situation.

### Rights and Needs of the Patient

The strength for coping with his disease rests within the patient himself; the caregiver's task is to help him discover and use that strength. The caregiver can ease the patient's fears and uncertainties and maintain the relationship the patient is asking for by listening to what the patient says or leaves unsaid about his diagnosis and prognosis. The patient's changing adaptive patterns can be translated into how, when and from whom he needs support. The physician who maintains close ties with his patients may be able to reach out and offer comfort; however, if in his judgment this service should be offered by someone else, he can call in a professional counselor either in the hospital or in the community. He may also be aware that troubled relatives often can talk with less embarrassment or guilt to a professional person not directly involved in the patient's medical care.

Paradoxically, while such counseling services are available and acceptable to low-income patients and their families through the large networks of hospital social service departments and community and welfare agencies, they are rarely considered an integral part of the total health care services provided to middle- and upper-income groups. Private patients and their families may not even know of the existence of counseling services or, if they do, may assign a stigma to them. "Social services are for welfare families," they may think. Or they may regard turning to

---

*A. D. Weisman, and T. P. Hackett, Predilection to death: death and dying as a psychiatric problem. *Psychosom Med, 23*:232-256, 1961.

professional help in a period of crisis as a sign of intolerable weakness. Sensitive to the prejudices of their private patients, physicians frequently are reluctant to suggest a resource which they would consider unsuited to their own status. As a result, the private patient and his family are left to cope with their problems in isolation.

For the caregivers, knowledge of what to anticipate, how to plan and to whom to turn for the different supportive measures called for throughout the period of illness should go a long way toward dispelling the anxiety, frustration and loneliness that are often generated by the disease. When the patient is accepted as he is, or even as he may become, then the supportive measures required for his care can be offered in an atmosphere of mutual respect and trust.

## The Family as Patient

While the needs of the patient are the primary concern of the medical team (and rightly so), the family is a kind of patient also. They, too, experience feelings of anger, guilt, loneliness and fear of rejection. Virtually every cancer patient that I have observed becomes more and more dependent on his doctor as his disease progresses. He moves away from formerly close relationships with his family, taking his doctor with him. While necessary for the patient's adjustment to his situation, this reaction often has a devastating effect on the member of the family who gives the most care and support. He himself has a need for direction and affection from the patient.

Although I continue to be deeply moved by the plight of the patient, I believe that the family, particularly the one who is most responsible for care, also should be given the opportunity for counseling. He should understand his own emotional stance in treating this particular illness. For while the patient can call on or be encouraged to ask for help from the doctor, nurse, social worker or chaplain if he needs help, members of the family frequently hesitate to reveal their own needs. Sometimes they are unwilling to burden the busy professionals with their problems, but are unaware of what resources are available to them.

The effect on the most dedicated family caregivers of being closed off both from medical personnel and, in some cases, from the patient himself, is a matter of deep concern. I believe, therefore, that the goal of treatment, especially when the disease has become hopeless, should not only be to provide optimum care of the patient but also to recognize when those caring for him need support and comfort.

Many patients and their families do not need help beyond medical and nursing treatment. They follow through with treatment and emerge from this life-threatening experience with a satisfactory mental and physical outlook. Often, however, treatment is blocked because the caregivers do not understand fully their complicated and demanding roles. If they become insecure and defensive, they can adversely affect the emotional climate of all concerned and even the well-being of the patient. How the family reacts plays a large part in prolonging the patient's life.

Therefore, the medical team not only must clarify the medical picture but, equally important, must help patients and their families identify and share the attitudes and reactions which are keeping treatment from being as good as it can be. The doctor's judgment becomes particularly important in considering the circumstances of the principal family caregiver. Although he and the other members of the health team can and do offer understanding and support of the family's difficulties, there may be times when a physician will notice signs of distress in a family member that can signal loss of control. Then he can recommend counseling from the same sources that are available to the patient.

RUTH D. ABRAMS

*15 Fairgreen Place*
*Chestnut Hill (Brookline),*
*Massachusetts*

# CONTENTS

NOT ALONE
WITH CANCER

# CHAPTER 1

# THE LOCALIZED STAGE
# (STAGE 1)

EACH diagnosis, whether of cancer or any other illness, may activate some preconceived ideas about the disease which are shared by many persons, and each individual patient, of course, reacts to the given diagnosis according to his own personality pattern. That cancer is a particularly life-threatening disease is generally conceded. To add to the insecurity created by this illness is the fact that, more frequently than in any other disease, the physician hesitates or questions, "How should I cope with this situation? What does the patient want to be told?"

Secretiveness has been lessened in recent years especially when the patient asks a direct question in a localized stage. Often the doctor's own anxiety magnifies the patient's fears and probably accounts for much of the restraint of professional helpers and of the family in dealing with the patient himself. The need for skillful clarification and emotional support cannot be stressed too much. Skill is also needed to determine what the illness means to the patient. The illness itself has a symbolic meaning, and in addition the medical procedures may change the patient's image of himself.

An added complication results when different persons tell the patient different things, or possibly when the patient unconsciously distorts what has been said. Thus, all who come in contact with the patient, especially the medical and paramedical personnel, should develop counseling skills with which they as well as the patient are comfortable.

If we accept the hypothesis that the patient is often aware of the fact that he has cancer and is reacting to that fact, whether he

3

says so or not,* we shall recognize the need for offering service which will afford better treatment and greater freedom from suffering. And again, if we believe that in cancer, as in any other illnesses, the mental attitude of the patient is a clue to understanding him and his family, we shall appreciate the need for further study of the reactions of these patients to diagnosis and treatment.

### Discovery of the Cancer Symptom

The discovery of the cancer symptom is usually made in one of two ways — by the individual himself or by a physician in routine examination. The patient reacts to finding the cancer with fear that the "lump," "wart" or "tumor" might be found "to be serious," "that thing I always dreaded" or "that thing my aunt died of."

Discovery is the first crisis for the cancer patient. If he discovers the symptom himself, he should report it immediately to his physician. Depending on the circumstances, the physician will ask the patient to come in for an examination or refer him to a specialist or clinic. If the patient has no physician of his own, he can ask his local hospital or medical society for a recommendation. Or he can go to the outpatient or emergency ward of a reputable hospital where he will either be seen immediately or will be referred for further examination.

If the symptom is found by a physician, he immediately recommends further examination to verify the significance of the symptom.

In either case, prompt evaluation of the symptom will help relieve the patient's uncertainty. If the symptom is nonmalignant, he will find relief for his anxiety; if it is malignant, he can benefit from immediate treatment.

### Phenomenon of Delay

All those who find for themselves a possible sign or symptom of

---

*J. E. Finesinger, H. C. Shands, and R. D. Abrams, Managing the emotional problems of the cancer patient. *Clinical Problems in Cancer Research—Sloan-Kettering Seminar,* Memorial Hospital, New York, 1951.

cancer go through phases of emotional reactions that are strikingly uniform. The one difference is in the timing of the phases; intervals between one phase and the next can range from minutes to years.

Almost every individual who finds a *danger signal* first thinks that it might be "a cancer," then quickly rationalizes his fears: "It couldn't happen to me." "This could not be cancer because there has never been any cancer in my family." "I have never been hit there." "I have no pain." "I have done nothing to deserve this." Then he puts it out of his mind, avoiding, suppressing or denying its possible significance. He "forgets all about it." Or does he? Actually, he retains some subconscious concern about the sinister implications of the symptom. He handles the concern in one of two ways: He seeks medical examination promptly or he delays.

The cause of delay in seeking medical examination of a possible cancer symptom has never adequately been identified. The delay and nondelay groups are statistically the same. However, it has been found in many studies, including the one I participated in at the Harvard School of Public Health,* that delay is not due to lack of knowledge of the seven danger signals, lack of funds, lack of time, lack of familiarity with available resources or even personal experiences with cancer. Many persons delay even when they suspect that the symptom means cancer and know that the chance of cure is better if they are treated early. As one medical educator wrote to a colleague, "I had pain in my stomach off and on for the past several months — but you know how it is — I kept putting off going to see a doctor. I knew all the time what he'd find."

The delayer is frequently heard to run through the reasons why it could not be cancer, but so do the nondelayers. It is not until the patient either notices a change in the symptom or finally confides in a friend that the delay is broken. The nondelayer is usually the individual who communicates easily with someone close to him, or even more important, who has a good relationship with a particular physician.

Perhaps the fact that cancer is the most dreaded disease is the most significant cause of delay. How can one expect an individual

---

*R. D. Abrams, Reasons for delay in seeking medical attention for signs or symptoms of breast cancer, 1952, unpublished.

to go promptly for medical examination of a possible symptom of cancer if he is convinced that "cancer is a death sentence"?

There is also fear of the unknown: What will radiation or X-ray do to the body? A number of patients, including those with other diagnoses, dread anesthesia even more than surgery or X-ray. As one patient said, "I'm scared of gas and ether. When I had my appendix out, they threw that thing on my face; I'll never forget it." Or, as another patient put it, "The reason I'm afraid to go to sleep is that I'm afraid of dying."

People with death wishes are also apt to delay. A 58-year-old woman, for example, had a lifelong fear that her husband would die suddenly as his father had and leave her widowed. She broke four appointments with her gynecologist to determine the cause of her vaginal bleeding before the physician realized that she unconsciously viewed the possibility of cancer as an opportunity to die before her husband.

Some people use delay as a means of getting attention. These people have fundamental feelings of not being loved or loved enough and believe that if they become critically ill, more attention will be paid to them. Such a patient was the woman who reported that when she mentioned the lump to her husband, he said it was nothing. "You're always looking for things to be nervous about."

Another important reason for delaying is the patient's reluctance to communicate with those close to him because his complaints are met with hostility and distrust. Similarly, if a patient has had an unpleasant experience with physicians or was afraid of them as a child, he will hesitate to report his symptoms promptly. One patient was scolded when she called for an appointment because her masseuse advised it. "What does she know?" the physician scornfully asked.

On the other hand, patients who can talk easily to members of their family and their physician will usually take prompt action when they discover suspicious symptoms.

A married woman of fifty told me about her symptom of breast cancer in a routine interview prior to her examination by a doctor in the Tumor Clinic.

"You might begin by telling me how you happened to come here today," I said.

"Well, I understood that this hospital was tops so to speak in this particular ailment. I have a growth . . . I found it when I finished bathing. I was just drying myself and this lump was in my breast. I'm conscious of things like that because it's been in my family. Probably my unconscious mind has caused me to be on the lookout for such things. So inasmuch as I understood that this hospital is so fine in this line, immediately on discovering this, I called up and made an appointment. I have all the confidence in the world in their being able to do something for me now that I have taken care of it in time. That's the way I feel about it. I haven't the slightest fear."

Many people suspect that lack of funds or the specter of the high cost of medical care is why patients delay. My studies show little evidence that this is the prevailing cause. Most patients with cancer symptoms realize that no physician or clinic will turn them away for lack of financial resources.

If the patient says he has a lump, a sore that will not heal, unusual bleeding, a nagging cough or a mole that is changing size, he will be seen. These are five of the seven common danger signals; the others are unusual bleeding or discharge, as from the rectum or vagina, and difficulty in swallowing (or indigestion).

It is discouraging that the number of delayers has not been significantly reduced despite widespread publicity about the symptoms and need for prompt treatment. There are instances where publicity appears to cause the person to be so frightened that he cannot talk about his symptom to anyone or take the advice that he knows all too well is essential. As one delayer said, "The magazines, radio, and TV make you so lump conscious . . . Last month there was this article in a women's journal about breast cancer. What I remember is that all those who went to the doctor within six months after noting the symptoms are alive today; all those who waited more than six months are dead . . . The article made me feel worse."

Although it is important to inform people about cancer, I am convinced that creating fear is not the answer to diminishing the delay period. Furthermore, I believe the word "victim" should not be applied to the cancer patient. What could be more fearsome than to be a victim of the most dreaded disease!

I have found that many delayers will finally seek help when they notice a change in the symptom. They may confide their concern to a friend or even a stranger, a nurse or a doctor who is treating a relative whom they are visiting. Or they may bring the symptom to the attention of their own physician just as they are leaving the office after consulting him about a different problem. I remember a man who was visiting his wife in the hospital and said to her doctor, just as he was leaving the room, "I wonder, Doc, if you could take a quick look at my neck. Something seems to be growing inside."

## Understanding the Delayer

Whether a patient delays or not carries strong implications for his progress in treatment. The patient who has not delayed comes to the clinic with the conviction that if it is cancer, because he has come *in time* he will be rewarded by a successful outcome. The doctor and other staff members share his attitude and accept and approve of him as a *good* patient. They stress that his treatment has the most chance of being effective.

But what about the delayer? He comes for initial examination with feelings of guilt. To become acceptable to the doctor in spite of his delay, therefore, he will, if given an opportunity, *confess* his delay to the doctor and others at great length. One such case was a 30-year-old woman I saw before she was examined by her doctor.

> "Back in July," she began, "I felt the lump in my left breast, and naturally the minute I felt it, I thought, as everyone does, of cancer. I went within a week to see my doctor. He said it was a blockage of one of the glands, and I should come back in a few months. I realize it has been more than a few months, but my father passed away and so many things happened . . . Anyway, last week I noticed an itchy feeling and it pained a little when I pushed on it and I felt a very small lump there. So my husband took me right up to the doctor again, and he gave me some medication and said if it didn't clear up I should go to the hospital. So, well, I'm here today."

No matter how realistic or unrealistic his excuses may be, this is the time when each caregiver should refrain from revealing disapproval of the patient. If the physician, especially, or other caregivers, including family members, display anger because the patient delayed seeking medical help sooner, then they will add to the patient's burden of guilt to the point where further examination and treatment may be blocked.

Instead, the physician or caregiver should listen to the patient and acknowledge his difficulties in coming for examination. It helps if the doctor indicates that many others have found it hard to seek medical attention for symptoms about which most people have fears. Such sympathetic acceptance can also help to relieve feelings of guilt which family members may harbor because they did not know of the symptom sooner or did not insist that the patient come immediately for medical examination. If the patient is helped to express his disturbing fears and feelings to an authoritative figure who understands him, he will tend to follow through with prescribed treatment promptly.

*Treatment*

Treatment of the localized cancer usually involves one or a combination of the following procedures: (1) surgical excision of the tumor, (2) implantation of radium to the site of the lesion and (3) X-ray therapy. Hospitalization is required for surgery or implantation of radium; X-ray therapy may be performed on an ambulatory basis in a hospital clinic or doctor's office.

X-ray and radium treatment can cause burning at the site, nausea and tiredness. Surgical removal of organs or limbs may require prosthetic devices to enable the patient to function at his optimum level.

When the patient presents himself for the first examination, the physician will usually recommend that the patient return to him or go to a specialist for testing of the affected area as an aid to verifying the diagnosis. A biopsy (a piece of tissue taken from the affected area for pathological testing) may be performed or X-rays taken. The doctor will not make a diagnosis until the results of the tests have been returned to him. If the patient is reluctant to go for further examination, however, he may have to be warned that it "could be a cancer" and that the only way to tell is by making the necessary tests.

### Telling the Patient

Once the diagnosis of cancer has been verified, the formerly healthy person suddenly becomes a person sick with a dreaded disease. Usually the physician will tell the patient that he has "cancer" or "a bad tumor" in a compassionate, yet straightforward, manner. The interview will be face-to-face in the doctor's office or at the hospitalized patient's bedside. Rarely will the physician impart such information on the telephone or by mail. A relative is included in the meeting only with the patient's permission. The patient usually either asks directly or indicates a wish to know the truth, often adding that he has always discussed his problems with one or more family members. This truthful interchange at this early stage is more and more becoming routine practice.

When necessary, it is the physician's responsibility to help the patient ask for his diagnosis. Even when, as often happens, a relative begs the doctor not to tell the patient his diagnosis, the physician must determine what is best for each patient and decide for himself what he believes the patient really wants to know. How well this procedure can work is illustrated by the following story.

> Helen Smith, forty years old, had had a wide excision for fibrosarcoma of the hip. For this type of cancer the outlook is generally poor. She came to my office after her one-year follow-up and said, "I've just seen Dr. W. and he says that I'm fine, that there is no evidence of cancer." I must have shown my surprise that she used the word cancer, because I recalled that her parents had made the surgeon promise not to tell her the truth. Her life had been difficult and they did not want to burden her with a new calamity.
>
> Helen went on to say that several months earlier, when she had asked Dr. W. why surgery had been performed, he told her the truth, that she had had cancer but he thought he had removed all of it. She asked him why he had not told her before. He told her of his promise to her parents. But now, he said, he could no longer lie to her. She was his patient, not her parents.
>
> Helen could understand her parents' point of view, but nevertheless was grateful to Dr. W. To this day, fifteen years later, she considers Dr. W. "the best doctor in the world and my best friend."

For some patients there are good reasons for tempering or withholding the facts. One is the patient who, in the physician's judgment, is too mentally or emotionally unstable to bear the truth. In his case, the physician will make sure the diagnosis is known to a responsible individual close to the patient.

Others from whom information should be withheld are those patients who repeat, both before and after the diagnosis, "If I have something bad, I don't want to know about it," or "I'm so afraid, I don't want to know the report of the findings." In spite of their conscious denial of their condition, however, these patients do follow through with treatment.

The decision regarding what to tell the patient should never be based on what the physician himself would want to know in his own case. Overidentification with the patient can have a detrimental effect on the doctor-patient relationship and hinder the patient's ability to follow through with treatment. I remember a distinguished consultant who after seeing a 32-year-old man with a form of cancer of the lymph glands said to the internist who had referred the patient, "He seemed like such a sensible fellow I told him the truth. I said he has acute Hodgkin's disease and nothing more can be done for him." Then, aware of the internist's surprise at this handling of the situation, he added, "Well, that's what I'd want to be told if I had it."

## The Caregiving Team: The Physician

If rehabilitation is to begin at the moment the patient comes to the hospital, we should realize the importance of making a plan as early as possible. The plan is subject to change and is based on the sharing of information among the professional persons caring for the patient. In a hospital this includes the physicians, nurses and social workers and more and more the hospital or the patient's chaplain.

The physician heads the professional group charged with the total care of the patient. He is the captain of the team. All that he learns from the patient as well as additional information derived from nurses, social workers and family members aids him in his total treatment of the patient. And he must give his consent for any additional professional help which nurses, social workers or vocational counselors suggest.

In the first interview the physician attempts to define the present clinical problem and to see this problem in the setting of the patient's past history. He tries to accomplish this in such a way that if further medical or laboratory examination is required, the patient-physician relation will be good enough to win confidence and cooperation . . .

A planned conversational approach or "master of ceremonies" technique is the best safeguard against rambling on the one hand or tightening up on the other. The physician or his interviewer plans to obtain useful data on certain topics: the present illness, the past medical history, the behavior of the patient with the interviewer, the family history . . .

The most natural starting point in history-taking is the present illness. The patient must then be allowed to talk without interruption as much of the time as possible, and the interviewer must show real interest in what is being said. The less talking the interviewer has to do to maintain the pattern described, the more effective he is likely to be. A rough rule is always to talk less of the time than the patient, and the best interviewers talk not more than one-tenth to three-tenths of the time.*

## The Caregiving Team: The Nurse

The doctor's closest assistant is the nurse who is the professional person on the scene. In her daily eight-hour bedside care of the patient, or as supervisor of the floor, the nurse observes the patient's reactions to the physical and emotional trauma of medical and surgical treatment. She is in a position to recognize his need for dependency or his wish for independence. She frequently helps the physician decide when a patient is emotionally able to undergo surgical or other treatment. She is able to be the bearer of comfort to the troubled patient. Her simple remark, "It must be hard," or "I can see that this isn't easy for you," often will provide the patient with the permission which he needs and wants to discuss his fears and concerns. "Without robbing him of his dignity, the nurse is in effect telling the patient that he is not a complainer or a bore, but just a person in trouble."† The nurse also is the one who is most aware of how the patient reacts to other patients on the ward and to his family, and hence can help

*J. E. Finesinger, Medical history taking, San Fransisco, California, September, 1949, unpublished.

†V. Barckley, The crises in cancer, *Am J Nurs,* February 1967.

in the plans for discharge.

Virginia Barckley pays tribute to the nurse as follows: *

Nurses can be of enormous help to patients at the time of diagnosis. . . . The nurse is the one who knows not to expect too much of a patient at this time. . . . Believing that "to everything there is a season," she knows there is a time for grief and crying, and that patients often can't enter into treatment plans the day after diagnosis. They need an opportunity to express their despair or anger, if that is what they feel, and it is the nurse who must dispel the impression that only stoicism is acceptable.

. . . Since nurses are with patients for longer and more critical periods than are almost any other professional people, they are often most able to help reduce the impact of loss of a body part or a change in body function. To do this effectively, though, a nurse needs some lasting philosophy to sustain her through the long, hard struggle for life, and when her own feelings of inadequacy, revulsion and hopelessness intrude.

## The Caregiving Team: The Social Worker

The most available counselor in the medical setting is the clinic social worker. She is considered a member of the medical team and usually has a master's degree in social work, awarded for helping individuals or groups through a regulated course of study in an approved school of social work. (There are about fifty-two of these schools in the United States.)

The social worker's knowledge of the usual reactions to cancer helps her understand her own patient's attitude, and from this she can help determine the degree of support to be offered and the goals of rehabilitation.

The questions the social worker will ask herself include the following:

Did the patient delay? Why?

Does he put blame on himself for his disease?

What were the reactions and advice of those with whom he has discussed his symptoms?

Does he see his illness as affecting his economic and social

---

*V. Barckley, What can I say to the cancer Patient? *J Pract Nurs,* April 1964.

status? And what is his present financial and social situation?
From the first interview, does it appear that the patient can
probably accept the recommended treatment?

After the first interview the social worker has a good idea as to
whether her continued support will be needed. She is the member
of the medical team who, more than any other, can be called on at
any time for future planning, even in the advanced cases when the
hospital no longer offers readmission or care.*

Many people think of the social worker as a person who gives
advice on how to manage the financial aspect of the illness. If they
do not need such help, their first reaction is to reject the
suggestion that such a person can be useful. I believe that changing
the term "social worker" to "mental health counselor" would be a
giant step toward ensuring acceptance by health workers and by
the family. His help should include practical matters, to be sure,
but it goes well beyond that.†

### The Caregiving Team: The Chaplain

The hospital chaplain who makes rounds as he chooses, without
need for direct referral as in the case of the nurse and social
worker, can first determine the spiritual needs of the patient and
in addition become the counselor. More and more chaplains are
being trained to give both spiritual and emotional support to
people who are sick and frightened. Their help, like that of the
social worker, can continue both within and without the hospital
setting. Or the chaplain may refer the patient to an appropriate
minister or priest in the community.

Not all patients want counseling by a minister of another faith,
or even of their own faith. Conversely, many patients are glad to
talk to a minister of any faith, so long as he has conviction about
the spiritual side of life.

Within the hospital medical students, physical and occupational
therapists, secretaries, ward maids and male attendants, and
volunteers offer additional and invaluable support to the patient

---

*R. D. Abrams, Social casework with cancer patients. *Soc Casework, 32*(10):425-432,
December 1951.
†R. D. Abrams, the responsibility of social work in terminal cancer. In *Psycho-social
Aspects of Terminal Care* (New York, Columbia University Press, 1971).

and his family.

It should be remembered that it is the patient himself who chooses the caregivers he wishes to help with his social and emotional problems. Apart from the medical team, the most important members of the caregiving team are the family members, relatives, friends and coworkers: They provide the day-to-day support that frequently makes the difference in how the patient accepts his illness and treatment.

## Patient's Response to Diagnosis

The initial response to crisis is anger and rage. And what crisis could be more devastating than the threat to life! It was not unexpected to find in a research study of sixty cancer patients that fifty-six responded to their condition by directing anger at themselves or others.

These patients appeared to have a need to find a cause for their illness. The illness was their fault or it was someone else's fault. In fact, all but four of these patients spontaneously assigned responsibility for having their disease to their misdeeds or those of others. "My husband made too many sexual demands on me," one woman said. Another attributed her cancer of the breast to her child who struck her in anger. Sometimes the patient's relative holds another person accountable. Mothers, for example, frequently blame their sons-in-law for their daughters' cervical malignancy.

Sometimes heredity is blamed for the disease. "Your mother died of cancer and now she's given it to our son," one distraught father angrily told his wife. Another said the disease came from a fall or a blow. "I never would have cancer if my brother hadn't hit me in the head with a baseball when I was a little boy," one young man told the nurse.

Patients frequently are afraid that they will pass the disease on to others. An elderly man with cancer of the rectum feared that if he returned to his daughter's house, he would spread the disease to his small grandchildren. Another man recalled that he had contracted syphilis as a teenager and although he had been successfully treated, he was sure he had caused his wife's malignancy.

Cancer causes both men and women to worry that they will no longer be able to perform their function as breadwinners, homemakers, sexual partners and parents. In a random study of sixty-two women with pelvic cancer,* the great majority (58) were housewives having the responsibility of their homes, their husbands and their children. Many represented the pivot around which the home took shape. Taking from the wife or mother her normal duties presented threats to her role as housekeeper, wife and mother. Similar fears regarding his role are frequently expressed by a male patient with cancer of the genital organs.

Frequently, the patient worries more about the treatment than he does about the disease. When surgery that will alter the body image is prescribed, the patient often will be consumed with anxiety. A woman who has had a breast removed fears that the false breast will be obvious to all who look at her. She can hardly believe that any man will find her desirable as a sexual partner. There is the same feeling of repugnance at the idea of having to maneuver an artificial hand or leg.

A patient, man or woman, with a colostomy worries that there will be some telltale smell of fecal matter, even though the bag to catch the output from the artificial opening of the intestine is not detectable and there is no smell. As one doctor with cancer of the rectum said to me, "Well, after the operation I wondered whether I had had a colostomy . . . started to call the nurse . . . thought I'd wait . . . if I did, I did . . . but luckily no. The whole thing was not very pleasant."

This last brings to mind the importance of telling the patient what has been found and what has been done as soon as he becomes conscious. The surgeon should do this himself, if possible. Waiting to hear the worst can have a poor effect on recovery.

Sometimes a patient's fears are of such intensity that he may make excuses for not keeping an appointment, continually shift the dates of treatment or make appointments with one doctor after another for examination or consultation in order to avoid treatment.

---

*R. D. Abrams, Social service and cancer: study of 62 gynaecologic patients. *J Obstet Gynecol,* 50:571-577, November 1945.

One of the difficulties in dealing with such fears is that so little is known about the cause of cancer that it is not always possible to ferret out the truth. How can one say at this present time with any certainty, for example, that cancer is neither hereditary nor contagious when one can find in medical and popular journals references to research in these areas?

Unfortunately, studies about the possibility of hereditary factors and viral infections as possible causes of certain types of cancer, for example cancer of the breast and leukemia, too frequently get wide publicity before they have been proven one way or another. Cancer is news and some reporters give out information prematurely. Wherever possible, caregivers should dispel fears that are as yet unproven.

It is important for patients in many cases to express their fears openly as the first step in readjusting to their new life situation. The nurse or clinic social workers can help. The nurse can say, for example, "You're probably wondering if the treatment is going to make you feel sick," or "Many people are more afraid of the treatment than they are of the disease." Then the caregiver can explain what surgery will do and how X-ray and radium treatments destroy the *bad* cells.

The doctor should be informed when a patient has not followed through with further examination or treatment so that he can get in touch with the patient. Unless the patient has sought help elsewhere, the doctor sees him again or brings him to the attention of some person in the setting, a member of the family, or the nurse, clinic social worker, secretary or medical student.

If the doctor or one of the caregivers finds that the patient or his family has deep neurotic reasons for not following through with treatment, he may refer the patient to a psychiatrist. In my experience this has rarely been necessary.

## Caregivers' Response to Diagnosis

In every encounter with a cancer patient, each caregiver should be alert not only to the patient's needs and wishes and how they can be met, but also to his own reactions to the patient and his diagnosis. The caregiver who has a pessimistic approach to the treatment of cancer must evaluate his attitude honestly, discuss it, if necessary, with other members of the caregiving team and decide if he can truly be helpful to the patient. (Certainly, he should avoid transmitting his negative feelings to the patient.)

If a patient is cared for by a sister or daughter, for example, who shows that she can scarcely look at the sick person, the situation becomes tragic and should be changed at all costs. Occasionally this happens. When it does, the family caregiver should not be criticized for his feelings but should be helped to communicate them to the nurse or some other member of the professional team. Once the tensions associated with the patient's illness are brought to light, the relative usually can accept responsibility for the patient's care. If not, he should be replaced by a more willing person, either professional or nonprofessional.

## *Financial Arrangements*

For many people, finances are a realistic problem which has to be resolved early in planning for future treatment and care. Usually arrangements can be worked out by the hospital admitting officer, who knows about third-party payment plans such as Blue Cross and Blue Shield, Medicare, Medicaid or veterans benefits. Or the patient may carry other insurance such as a plan provided by the company for which he works. The admitting officer also can help the patient apply for and accept public welfare medical aid such as disability assistance, when this is appropriate.

Many patients expect that funds are available from the hospital or other private resources; however, this is rarely the case and that fact should be explained immediately to the patient.

## *Response to Treatment Program*

In spite of the fear, anger and guilt that the patient may be suffering prior to treatment, rarely does he fail to follow through with treatment as planned. The fact that he usually appears on time for the prescribed treatment, with a minimum of prodding by the physician, paramedical personnel or family members, suggests his real awareness of the medical situation and his wish to have something done.

The physician selects the type of treatment he believes affords the best chance for the arrest or cure of the disease. The patient and his family need to know beforehand what treatment has been prescribed and they should have the opportunity to learn why a particular type of treatment or program has been recommended. It is the patient's and family's prerogative to ask questions and, whether or not there is a choice, to discuss their feelings about the type of treatment they prefer or had in mind.

The patient must have faith in the physician's choice of treatment plan. Here, again, it must be emphasized that the doctor, the patient and the family need to feel that they have formed a partnership whose goal is the patient's recovery. The doctor must have the confidence of both the patient and his family.

When the treatment procedures are completed, the physician tells the patient as soon as possible that the "cancer," "bad tumor" or "bad cells" have been eradicated and that the diagnosis and prognosis are optimistic. The physician and other caregivers should take the time to discuss the patient's concerns about the effects of the treatment and the readjustments that may be necessary. The patient should be told honestly about the chances for recurrence of the disease and the need to report to his physician for periodic re-examination.

It is not necessary, however, to tell the patient more than he needs to know or to alarm him unduly about what might have happened. As one patient said, "I was glad the doctor told me the truth after the removal of my breast — that I had cancer — but I was frightened when he added that it had not spread. I never thought of *that.*"

## Discharge from the Hospital

The discharge from the hospital comes as both a shock and a relief for the patient and his family. If the patient becomes unusually angry, depressed or afraid to return home, the medical team personnel should consider further probing focused on the patient's possible shame or disgust with changes in body image brought about by treatment.

The patient often needs the opportunity to understand his own anger in order to regain freedom of communication with members of his family. In addition, the family may need to be singled out by the nurse or social worker for help with their adjustment to the changes in the patient's physical image. In other words, the patient needs to learn first from the medical personnel and then from his family that there is nothing about his illness, the effect of treatment or his reactions which cannot be understood and handled. Acceptance of the patient as he now is and will be helps him to regain confidence in himself and in those close to him.

If a patient requires a prosthesis, he should be given ample opportunity to reveal his anxieties about using it. One helpful program is the one organized by the American Cancer Society for cancer patients who have just undergone mastectomies. Volunteers who have themselves had a breast removed visit the patients in the hospital to discuss such practical matters as being fitted properly for a false breast, as well as the emotional issues associated with loss of body image. Group therapy can also be helpful for people who must learn to cope with a colostomy.

Following treatment, most people in the initial stage can take care of themselves and resume their former occupations. If not, they should be helped to plan for a reduced program more in keeping with their capabilities. With the patient's consent, employers, teachers, family members, lawyers, insurance agents and others who are directly involved can be given a truthful explanation of the patient's condition by a professional caregiver. Then they can accept him better and help him resume his old activities or readjust to new ones. The clinic social worker can arrange for physical and vocational rehabilitation services and continuing counseling. When a patient returns home, he should be viewed as one who has been sick but is recovering and adjusting to the best of his ability. The atmosphere to which he returns should be hopeful and constructive.

If, following discharge, the patient requires only minimal care, he can usually manage with a relative or friend to assist him. But if he needs skilled nursing services, such as replacing numerous dressings or daily colostomy irrigation, he probably should have the help of a visiting nurse, who usually can help the family take over the patient's care. It is a good plan for visiting nurses to have an opportunity to participate in the nursing procedures while the patient is still in the hospital. Personally, I believe some family member should also share this experience before the patient leaves the hospital.

Patients who cannot return to their family settings immediately can be placed in an appropriate convalescent home. However, in my experience this is necessary in only a few situations, usually when patients are a long distance from home. Even men who live alone have returned to their one-room apartments where a landlady helped give them the care they needed.

When there is no other alternative, however, the patient and his family should be helped to accept the realistic need for nursing home placement.

## *Follow-up*

The follow-up period can cover a span of weeks, months or years during which the patient returns at regular intervals for medical examination. Immediately following the initial treatment, he exhibits changes in behavior and pattern of communication. At the clinic or doctor's office, as he awaits his examination, he seldom expresses the fear and anxiety he feels, yet his uneasiness is apparent. He is strangely quiet and remote. He rarely talks with other patients or personnel with whom he had previously spoken freely. Once the physician tells him that he has found "no new lump," he escapes from the clinic as soon as possible. In fact, he leaves so hurriedly that the medical team has no opportunity to evaluate his progress socially, emotionally or vocationally.

My observations have led me to believe that this marked change simply means that the patient does not want to be reminded of his illness and the many ways in which it threatens his continued existence. He is practicing a form of denial, wishing to banish the disease by banishing all acknowledgment, except the necessary medical one, that it ever happened to him. Cancer, he seems to be saying, is not a matter for general conversation as is frequently the case in other illness situations.

## Clues to Helping the Patient

I believe that whatever means of coping a patient uses to maintain himself in a very difficult and painful illness should be respected. A patient who is managing to carry on daily activities without causing distress to himself or those who are close to him probably does not require interventive services. However, the doctor, nurse and social worker must know enough about the patient's adjustment to determine when additional services and emotional support are needed by the patient and his family. They should be especially alert to maladaptive patterns of coping which may have a disruptive effect on good professional and family relationships.

One patient who had had a mastectomy, for example, came to me in the middle of the summer wearing a heavy coat. "Do you feel you have something to hide?" I asked. She then told me that she felt ashamed at being "lopsided" and had been too embarrassed to be fitted for a false breast. I was able to help her accept her situation and to make the necessary arrangements for her fitting.

Another patient, a 45-year-old man, had failed to go back to work following the amputation of his leg. He was reluctant to return to the department store where he had been a floor manager, a job which required that he be on his feet most of the day. I was able to persuade the patient to talk freely with his former employer about the nature of his operation. The employer transferred him to the accounting department, where he was able to perform a useful service without having to stand up all day.

Thus, although during the follow-up period the patient is retreating from the fact of having cancer and from the professionals who were associated with his illness, the caregivers should stand ready to revive the partnership with the patient that was effective at the time of treatment. The patient would thus be assured that the physician and those closest to him continue to be interested in him as a person with a future.

The following story is typical of the optimism about the illness and of the planning ahead which most cancer patients describe in the recovery from initial treatment. This letter, written by a psychiatrist, Dr. C., who had had surgery for a malignant tumor of the stomach, was written to a friend and colleague:

> I do want to let you know that I'm officially and unofficially postconvalescent. I'm really feeling ever so much better. Have gained back a few pounds and am working along fairly well. It's good to be back in circulation again even though a few cylinders are a bit wacky.
>
> About three months or so ago I had some lower abdominal pain — eventually a barium enema and a diagnosis of diverticulitis [pouchings in the intestinal tract]. You know the doctors and their problems. The professor down here decided to take a look and told me he found a "neoplasm" [malignancy] which he got completely — so if he thinks so I'll agree. My surgeon's anxiety was pretty evident when on the day of the operation he asked, "Well, Bill, how did you sleep last night?" To which I replied, "More important, how did *you* sleep?" Actually, I'm much better and believe one could write a couple of volumes on the doctors and their anxiety.
>
> This whole experience has convinced me all the more that it's good to be able to talk about CA, speaking with the family and some others, too. So I've made many good resolutions, most of which I left at the hospital. I've been staying home and being a good ex-patient. I'm still planning to go to Europe for some army teaching in a few months.

Later, this same individual admitted some frustrations due to the reactions of those around him once he had returned to work. I believe the majority of cancer patients have had similar embarrassing experiences with colleagues and friends. As Dr. C. told it: "A doctor I know well met me at a meeting. He said nothing, so I said to him, 'How do *you* feel, *I'm* fine.' " Dr. C. added, "So many people can't look at me, even at staff meetings."

These remarks give us food for thought. Instead of looking away, we must give the cancer patient returning from the first treatment the opportunity to answer questions about his illness, just as we would any other patient.

For increasing numbers of cancer patients, the story of their illness ends here. Although they continue to return for periodic reexamination, their cancer does not recur and after a long period in which no new symptoms appear, they are guardedly considered *cured.* The best means of helping such a patient to feel that he remains in control of his life is to maintain the atmosphere of

optimism  and  show  concern  for  his  emotional  as  well  as  physical
recovery.

# CHAPTER 2

# REGIONAL INVOLVEMENT
# (STAGE 2)

$\mathrm{T}$HE case of Raphael Martino, an attractive, 19-year-old single man of Italian descent, comes to my mind when the stage of cancer known as "regional involvement" is being described. I first met this young man when readmission to the hospital was recommended for treatment of a mass in his left groin. Eight months previously his left undescended testicle had been removed when a diagnosis of cancer was confirmed.

Raphael was understandably upset. He directed his anger at everyone, probably because he had not been cured and was frightened that recurrence was evident. He was especially fearful at the prospect of telling his mother the threatening news. At the time of my interview it appeared that I could be helpful by offering to drive him home and telling his mother, which he readily accepted.

During the trip there was an outpouring of his fears. He asked about his illness. "What do I have? Can you tell from the record what I have got?" At first, I kept the subject on the treatment for the tumor in the groin. I repeated that the doctor said it must be treated by surgery to get rid of it. Raphael said that he believed he had the disease people fear most. Then he went on to add that people should be told what they have. The doctor only said that he had found another tumor like the one in his testicle. "If I am very ill, I can take it. If it is meant to be it will be. Tell me really, what sense is there in operating if in the end the disease cannot be stopped? I will not permit an operation if it is hopeless. Why go through all this. It was bad enough having a testicle removed — it is awful!

Raphael sobbed and repeated that he could not face telling his mother. She would be so upset. Dr. Smith had assured him in the beginning that the groins were not involved. He had had such terrible dreams about coming back to the hospital. Someone was always chasing him and he could not escape. He was afraid this would happen. Oddly enough, he had had to come back here with his mother, who recently had had a hysterectomy, and again to see a friend of his father. He could not seem to get away. Consciously he thought he would not have to come back except for checkups. He had never given it a thought, but subconsciously he guessed he was scared. He had hoped he would have Dr. Jones, the doctor he had had and liked so well before; however, now he hoped Dr. Moore, the chief, would do the job.

Raphael then said that although it was a bad day, it was a beautiful world. A year ago all had been well. He had never been sick. Now look at him. His girl friend, who worked in the same place as he did, used to come to see him every day he was in the hospital. It was hard on her. No one would know he was sick. He had no pain. He was not tired. He wished he were like the gangsters. They were bad, but he would have traded with them any day. They had healthy bodies. If he had to have his other testicle removed, he wouldn't agree to that; no sir. How he hated to go back into the hospital. He was there six weeks the last time. He had not gone back to school after he was sick. His mother had needed some money, so he went to work. He was a clothes presser in a factory. He liked his work and wondered what he would do about it now.

He turned to me and said, "You've seen a lot of people like me up in that clinic. Am I reacting like the others?" "Yes, you are reacting just the way I would have expected you to do. It is awfully hard to reenter the hospital for more surgery when you've already had the kind of major surgery you had before."

Finally, the car stopped before a dilapidated house. "This," said Raphael, "is home. I wouldn't mind the operation so much if I could stay here to have it done."

His mother was washing dishes. She greeted me pleasantly. She did not seem to realize that it was unusual for me to have brought her son home. Her English was hard to understand. Without waiting, I explained the need for her son to have further surgery for a tumor found in his groin. After a few moments she seemed to grasp the significance of what I was saying. (Undoubtedly, she had been told by the surgeon at the time of operation that Raphael had cancer. In most hospitals it is policy for a doctor to tell the diagnosis to a responsible relative.) Thus, she undoubtedly grasped that the disease had spread. Mrs. Martino became hysterical and shouted to her son to go upstairs. Her conversation then centered around her troubles of being left by her husband seventeen years ago to face the difficulties of her own health. She could not and would not do it any longer. She stood holding her head and swaying. I agreed that it was very hard for her, but that it was perhaps hardest for her boy.

Suddenly, Mrs. Martino regained her control, calling her son to come downstairs. Before he returned she added, "In my heart I cry, to my son I smile." Putting her arm around the boy, she said, "Well, I guess you have to do what the doctor says. We'll be good soldiers, won't we, son? We have before."

This is one of the ways in which regional involvement comes to light, and the reaction of mother and son is normal. I kept in close contact with both of them throughout the second hospital admission, offering specific services when he returned home and helping to clarify the medical situation.

There are times when the cancer has reached the stage of regional involvement at the time of first medical examination. The patient may or may not have delayed, or the delay might have been unavoidable. This was true for Mrs. Anna Pappas, a tense, ambitious Greek Orthodox woman of thirty-eight who knew for months before coming to this country with her ailing husband, son and daughter that she had a mass on her hip. She had sought no previous examination in Greece and told no one of her findings for fear that something would interfere with the approval of her long-awaited visa to the United States.

Mrs. Pappas's chief concern following referral for hospital admission for probable surgery was how her illness would affect the plans she had for her son to go to medical school, her daughter to a school of nursing and for herself to help manage a small family business owned by her husband's relatives.

When amputation of the leg because of fibrosarcoma of the hip (a high-risk type of cancer) was recommended as the only means of saving her life, her screams of despair and fear could be heard all over the hospital. However, she regained control of herself remarkably quickly. By the time I reached her side later in the day she was full of questions, such as: Would she be able to wear an artificial limb? How much did they cost? How would she arrange payment? I was able to assure her on all counts. The doctors said she could be fitted for a limb, she could in time learn to walk with crutches, and the artificial leg could be paid for partially by a fund in the hospital for prostheses. The remainder she would pay whenever she was able. This was all discussed during the days prior to amputation and afterward. She did experience a period of depression following surgery, but quickly managed the crutches and the temporary limb. At home she continued her progress with the aid of her daughter, the visiting nurse and the physical therapist. Soon she was able to resume household activities to a limited degree. Her in-laws paid for many household expenses. They, as well as the patient herself, were against accepting from Public Welfare's Disability Assistance.

Frequently, in our interviews during follow-up visits she referred to a sin committed years ago. She considered that she was being punished for this sin. Finally, one day I said, "What was this sin you talk about so frequently?" To which she replied that when she was pregnant with her third child in Greece she had taken a pill which caused a miscarriage one month later. Although she understood realistically that there was no reason to believe that the pill itself could have been the cause of her losing this baby, she did have thoughts that God had punished her for her evil idea and deed. I suggested that she seek out her priest, and she asked me to do this for her. I gave the priest no details, but only stated her medical situation and that she wished to see him. Following several interviews with this clergyman, her feelings of guilt subsided somewhat and this probably helped her toward a reluctant acceptance of her illness and the loss of her limb.

Actually, Mrs. Pappas was most successfully rehabilitated. Although she did not help in running her relatives' store, I did arrange for her to work full-time in the sewing room of the Massachusetts General Hospital. A neighbor provided transportation and Mrs. Pappas has continued in the job for ten years. Her children, although not becoming doctor or nurse, continued their higher education to the satisfaction of their mother. Every year Mrs. Pappas, who had regional involvement, telephones me after her annual checkup to report the good news of "no recurrence."

## The Cancer Spreads to Adjacent Areas

Cancer is considered to have reached the stage of regional involvement (Stage 2) when the disease has spread to nearby adjacent areas or contiguous structures in the body and is found microscopically to be of the same type of malignancy as the original lesion.

The doctor may have found the tumor in the adjacent area at the time of routine checkup of the original lesion, as in the case of Raphael, who was unaware of the mass in his groin until it was found by the doctor to have spread from the original site. Or the disease may have reached Stage 2 at the first examination if there was delay, as in the case of Mrs. Pappas.

At this stage, the outlook is fair to guarded — no longer good, as it was in the localized stage. The medical treatments that follow may arrest or even cure the patient or prolong his life for months or even years. If, unfortunately, the patient's disease metastasizes (spreads to other parts of the body beyond the original site or parts adjacent to it), then the disease enters the advancing, usually hopeless, stage.

The localized stage comes abruptly to an end when symptoms of invasive regional involvement are identified. In other words, Stage 2 presents far more problems for the patient, his family and the professional personnel than did the localized stage. Now the outlook is cautious, less optimistic. The patient and his family are aware consciously or unconsciously that the goal of treatment is to stop the disease from spreading to other organs. There begins to be a closure in the free and honest communication of the preceding stage. Too suddenly, it becomes clear to all involved, including the patient, that earlier treatment has not eradicated the disease or that even on this first visit the disease has already spread locally to nearby areas.

*Telling the Patient and His Family*

After determining by biopsy, X-ray or surgery that the new mass or growth is cancerous and of the same type as the primary lesion, the doctor usually conveys his findings to the patient with more guarded honesty than in the initial stage. "I guess we've found a bit of the old trouble," or "I'm afraid we have to treat this 'growth,' 'tumor' or 'cancer' as we did the first one." To the family he speaks with candor. "The cancer has spread to another nearby part of the body and we must do something about it."

*Treatment*

Surgery, radiation or radium, or a combination of one or more of these procedures, may be applied to the lesion. When indicated, varying forms of chemotherapy are administered, orally or intravenously, to destroy or arrest the cancer cells. Drug administration requires close medical supervision. The type of drug can be altered for the effect on or comfort of the patient; it may produce nausea and excessive fatigue, but these gradually disappear.

Emotionally, the regional involvement stage is an extremely trying time for everyone, especially when the patient has already been treated and the disease has recurred. The patient, his family, the physician and everyone who has taken part in his care is overwhelmingly disappointed. The patient and family are angry with the medical team for having let them down. Perhaps they feel guilty that they did not do all they could to find "a better doctor." The medical team harbor feelings of anger that recurrence has come too soon, and they may question whether some other type of medical procedure, or some additional type of therapy could have been more effective. These disappointments rarely are expressed, but frequently they are felt by all concerned.

As a senior surgeon at a well-known clinic said, "Although I have been operating upon patients with cancer for thirty-six years, I still have a feeling of defeat whenever I cannot remove all the tumor and so cure the patient." He added that this defeatist attitude is not helpful when it comes to subsequent care of the patient. From this point on, all are faced with an uncertain future in which the pendulum may swing toward victory or defeat, hope or despair. Quite evidently, the partnership between the patient and his doctor and the patient and his family is threatened because communication has reached a new and bewildering stage.

We recognize at this point that cancer is different from other diseases. Its most significant and frustrating feature is that, except for reporting to his physician, the patient has no control over his disease at this or any other stage — at least as far as we know today. This is unlike the case of a patient with heart disease who through rest and medication frequently stabilizes his illness, or the diabetic patient who may control his disease through diet and insulin. The patient with cancer sees his disease as a purely medical one whose progression cannot be altered by control of physical or emotional activity or by renouncing excesses of any kind. Cancer may recur, spread or even disappear at any time.

There are both positive and negative aspects to this helplessness. On the one hand, the patient's activities can be continued without influencing the disease process adversely; on the other hand, not being able to present himself as the *good* patient becomes a subtle but significant deterrent to the doctor-patient relationship. In short, the inability to play the real part in managing the disease process influences both the patient and his physician, especially at this stage of the illness.

## Patient's Defensive Denial

Despite the uncertainties of the medical situation and the mutual feelings of anger, guilt and frustration, the patient, his family and the medical team feel a strong need to have something done. The physician's anxieties about the case are somewhat alleviated once he prescribes a new treatment program. His explanation to the patient that the new treatment has a good chance of arresting the disease permanently, or at least for a period of time, offers some comfort and hope. The patient accepts the physician's plan for treatment with a minimum of questioning. But he cannot face realistically the new and frightening invasion of the disease to nearby areas. Often he begins to employ defensive emotional maneuvers, most notably avoidance and denial, to allow him to cope with his more uncertain situation. Unlike the earlier stage, now the patient does not want all the details of diagnosis, treatment and prognosis. Paradoxically, he may ask everyone in the setting but his doctor for clarification of his medical situation. He may even complain to others that the physician has not told him everything. Yet he seldom asks his physician directly for information about his condition, and if he does he rarely pursues the subject on subsequent visits. My data substantiate what physicians repeatedly state: In this period, patients do not want to discuss their illness with them. Further, most patients do not ask the physician about their medical status even when he makes a conscious effort to pave the way for them to do so. They employ such excuses as, "The doctor was so busy," or "He looked so tired." "There were so many other patients to be seen," or "I don't want to upset him because he has tried so hard to help me." When I suggested directly to a particular patient that he ask his physician for a true account of his medical condition, as he had often talked of doing, he said he preferred not to because "maybe those are questions I wouldn't want answered."

The occasional patient who did inquire of his physician usually said he wished he had not. As one patient put it, "The doctor told me too much — well, it wasn't too much, it was what I wanted to know, but I wonder if I really did — if I did the right thing."

Patients who formerly spoke directly about their medical situation and treatment now become amnesic about the course of the illness, focusing their attention on bodily symptoms or even suggesting that other possible pathological processes or other diseases are responsible for their symptoms. A 35-year-old mother of three with metastases to the spine from a carcinoma of the breast repeatedly said to her surgeon, with whom she had talked readily and honestly during the initial period, that she "would be worried only if what she had in her back was related to her former breast condition." She insisted that her pains were caused by arthritis, although she knew that her mother had died of similar complications after a mastectomy only three years previously.

When the surgeon asked me how he should meet her denial, I suggested that as long as the patient wanted him to avoid discussion of the truth, he should go along with her. In other words, this patient, like so many others, was telling the doctor what she herself wanted and needed to believe in order to cope with the situation. The patient's defense against the truth of threatening disease, which paradoxically does not usually disturb his acceptance of treatment or disturb any other area of his life, should in my opinion be accepted and respected. By avoiding open discussions with his physician about the reality of his situation, the patient may be better able to make plans and carry them out.

While the patient studiously avoids discussion of his diagnosis and prognosis, he will, however, talk freely about such safe matters as diet, daily regimen and symptoms. For example, a 48-year-old woman with metastatic ovarian cancer kept a list of questions for the physician at each appointment. Should she continue to take Bufferin® and douches? Should she walk more, bathe and so forth? She also discussed future plans, but she never mentioned the diagnosis and prognosis as she had in the initial period.

Diet, too, is a favorite subject. The following are excerpts of conversations which I heard one day as I sat in the waiting room of the X-ray therapy section. They illustrate how successfully the ill can bypass their real troubles. All the speakers were private patients with different types of Stage 2 cancer.

The first man who enters the room is a distinguished looking, 72-year-old father of a prominent minister who lives out of state and is staying at a nearby hotel during the course of X-ray therapy. He greets everyone affably and says that he is feeling pretty well. Soon after, a 56-year-old South American man of great wealth and sophistication arrives. He immediately starts to talk about his diet. He feels well and has no ill effects from the treatment and bases this on the fact that he has found out that the best thing to do is to limit himself to three meals a day. He directs his conversation to the 60-year-old gentleman from New York City who has just joined the group. The latter interrupts frequently to say that he has no appetite and finds eating difficult. The South American continues by passing around his diet list which he has written out in detail, saying that the last time he had treatment up here he ate between meals, and that took away his appetite for his big meals.

The pros and cons of eating certain foods are then discussed. The patient from New York says that he was told nothing about diet and eats as he pleases.

The South American turns to the New Yorker and says, "What do you do in your spare time? I have so much time I don't know what to do with myself." The man from New York says that he reads a lot and has many visitors, mostly women, who are making a terrible fuss over him. The South American welcomes my suggestion that if he is interested, there is good theater and music in Boston which I would be glad to direct him to. Aside from this, I have not taken any part in the conversations, nor were any remarks directed to me. I have not met these patients before, and there is no reason for them to know at this time that I am one of the staff.

The machine and how it works also figures in patients' conversation. When the amount of time under treatment is altered, the patient should be told the reasons by the radiologist or nurse; otherwise he may get a wrong idea about the effect of treatment. It should also be explained that different machines may be used at various times. That these machines often break down is also annoying and disturbing. Even being alone in a room with such a high voltage machine is frightening, but few patients express this unless asked directly.

The wise caregiver will take his clue from the patient. He will do his best to relieve disturbing preoccupations brought to his attention and will avoid focusing on the anxiety which the patient wishes to deny.

### Doctor-Patient Relationship

The initial frankness of the doctor-patient partnership now changes. One patient said, "When the doctor looked at my breast I saw the expression on his face and knew I had cancer. When I asked him what he thought it might be he fenced with me like in a play." The doctor does not want to alarm the patient by relating all the possibly grave details of his prognosis, and the patient withdraws more and more from confronting the true facts about his illness. Nor will the physician predict in detail the outlook for the patient's future, especially since he cannot do so with certainty. He realizes that too much explanation of the type of lesion, the rate and extent of its growth and the probable effect of the prescribed treatment can cause more confusion and anxiety for the patient and his family.

Another threat to the doctor-patient relationship is the need to call in specialists and consultants when the stage of regional involvement is reached. The patient is presented to more and more specialists for consultation and is told less and less about what is happening. He may be presented to a conference of doctors where, often, in complete disregard for his feelings, he hears differing opinions about the efficacy of various treatment methods. Angry and resentful at being depersonalized, the patient feels increasingly impotent and anxious about the outcome of any treatment. He begins to wonder "who my doctor is," and both he and his family suffer from the uncertainty of not knowing to whom to go for support. It is extremely important at this stage for the medical team to clarify who is the doctor in charge, both to relieve anxiety and to maintain the viability of the doctor-patient relationship.

When prepared, the patient's acceptance of a new doctor is usually less traumatic than might be expected. In a study of twenty-seven patients with Stage 2 cancer of the breast, the attending doctor was a young man who carefully spent much time and thought in talking to each patient about her present situation, including the diagnosis, the treatment and its possible effects. Before he left the institution, preparation for separation had been carefully worked through with each of his clinic patients by the physician and other members of the team. His place was taken by a female doctor who was equally careful and thoughtful, but by nature far less communicative and more restrained. The patients accepted her without noticeable tension, depression or alteration in their adjustment.

The importance of this observation was in contrast to that made by a psychiatrist at the same institution who noted that the neurotic patients whom he was similarly preparing for separation were experiencing considerably more emotional tensions and difficulties in maintaining their previous level of adjustment. This ability on the part of the cancer patient at this crucial period to accept change in his doctor, especially when prepared, is important because it enables a battery of personnel in different settings to accomplish the services required.

Paradoxically, the patient becomes less open but more dependent on the physician as the disease progresses. Haunted by a nagging fear of rejection, he becomes uncomplaining, *good,* passive, overly nice and overly cooperative. He will accept referral from one physician to another without complaint as change in treatment procedures becomes necessary. He makes no demands to be seen at the time of the scheduled appointment and will wait at the clinic for indefinite amounts of time without signs of impatience or resentment. He continues to deny the significance of the actual symptoms of recurrence, while convincing himself that the medical profession and science itself are omnipotent.

Aware that he is solely dependent upon therapy that only a physician can suggest or provide, he departs after each visit with only one hope: that the physician, any physician, will see him again. The return appointment signifies for him a confirmation of hope that there is still some treatment that might counteract the disease. Although this was not always true, today a patient is always given a return appointment either by the attending doctor or clinic secretary, or he will be referred elsewhere to a particular specialist, local family doctor or clinic for further follow-up. Thus, the patient is ensured of the continuation of regular medical care.

The patient regards the physician as the paramount figure in his life; all others assume a peripheral role. Rarely will he enter into discussions, as he did in the earlier stage, with the social worker, nurse, secretary or even the chaplain, nor does he want his family involved with the medical team. If possible, he comes to the clinic unaccompanied so that there will be no opportunity for his family to discuss the truth of his illness with the doctor or others. The patient is, in effect, limiting acknowledgment of his medical condition to his personal clinic visits, where he refuses to discuss the reality of his symptoms.

In the physician's presence he suppresses his fear and anger, saving it for those who have no direct responsibility for his medical care. "My doctor isn't giving me enough blood," one patient told me. Another complained that he was not getting the right sleeping pills. "If only my legs would improve," a client of mine sighed, "I'd be all right."

## Relationships with Family Caregivers

The caregivers, especially the family members closest to the patient, are hurt when the patient does not seem to need them. Frequently they must also bear the brunt of the patient's realistic fears and anxieties. When the patient turns away from them they become increasingly disturbed about their inability to help him.

If the family, friends, employer, teacher and others close to the patient can anticipate and understand the withdrawal, it may be easier for them to refrain from offering services which the patient does not want, yet remain available when needed again.

To help the family to accept the patient's changing pattern of behavior, the physician may initiate referral to a caregiver within or outside the hospital setting. To date, these services are rarely offered, yet they can be essential in helping to maintain the strength of the family, especially if irreversible disease is the next stage in the patient's illness.

## Rehabilitation and Follow-up

As in the localized stage, when the treatment is completed the patient should be encouraged to resume a program of activities in keeping with his maximum capabilities. He will return for periodic examinations to his physician or clinic and he will exhibit the same anxiety and the same denial and avoidance as he did formerly. The nurse, social worker or chaplain should reach out and suggest the necessary steps that should be taken whenever the patient and his family are having social, emotional or vocational difficulties which are interfering with the patient's life.

This was brought out in the case of Mrs. Pappas. When this patient appeared to need more support than had been offered, I encouraged her to share with me and her priest the sin to which she had repeatedly referred. I considered that the use of intervention at this point of obvious anxiety might clear up an area of concern which, if not discussed openly, would threaten her rehabilitation.

There are times in a person's life when respect for who he is and how and from whom he wishes help are more important than anything else.\* In the second stage of cancer, communication appears to be most in jeopardy, characterized by guarded attitudes and circumlocution. But, to one who can follow the clues, it is the most revealing stage of the illness. It is often through what the patient leaves unsaid or when and to what he may change the subject that the caregiver learns the areas of the patient's greatest anxiety, areas of definite taboo.

For the professional caregivers, who can give support in a variety of ways, it is difficult to accept the fact that there comes a time in the course of cancer when the patient no longer desires personal contact with anyone but his physician, and then only for medical treatment and not for emotional support. Perhaps the greatest change for the physician comes in accepting the omnipotence which the patient assigns to him. Usually, the nurse must be content with giving nursing care and the social worker with providing specific services.

The family and professional caregivers should concentrate on the strengths still in evidence in the majority of these patients. One of the most significant strengths is the patient's good relations with his physician. If a family or friend asks too many questions about the doctor and his treatment or alludes to the more favorable results of those treated by other doctors or methods, this may undermine the patient's confidence in his doctor and cause the relationship to deteriorate. Family and friends rarely know the patient's whole medical picture and are thus in no position to offer medical advice. They should concentrate on mending any reservations the patient may have about the doctor or treatment before the advanced stage is reached. If that stage never comes, so much the better.

The following letter from a prominent Boston minister was distributed to all his parishioners. He was suffering from Stage 2 cancer at the time. This patient knows and admits that his tumor is inoperable, yet he continues to hope that its growth can be arrested. He expresses the desire "to take some of the fear out of cancer," but his words, "some live, some die," imply fear of the

\*R. D. Abrams, and B. Dana, Social_work in the process of rehabilitation. *Soc Work,* October 1955.

disease and even fear of dying. There seems to be a preoccupation with ideas of helplessness and hopelessness, which perhaps as a minister he feels he should not express. He contradicts himself when he states on the one hand that "it helps just to be able to talk about it" and follows this with "right now, the less said or written to me about it, the better."

He also implies that his disease is his concern alone, that he wishes to manage it himself. He can be helped if others do not talk amongst themselves, "whisper," about his situation. This last appears almost naive in a man of his understanding of human nature, but it also reminds us that, regardless of profession or training, individuals all harbor similar fears of too much discussion in which they can take no part.

Finally the last paragraph sums up his fear and uncertainty about his future, while at the same time he shows his need for the love and compassion of his parishioners, who actually are the only family this particular man has.

My Dear People:

This is my first message to you since I was operated on two weeks ago tomorrow. The operation was an illustration of that mysterious fact of life: what we are looking for we often do not find, and what we do find is not what we are looking for.

So it was with the operation. The doctors found no trouble where they were looking for it. What they did find was a malignant tumor in the area of the gallbladder which was interfering with the normal flow of bile. They rerouted the bile so that it can now flow freely. The foreign body which they did not expect to find could not be removed, nor can it be treated by X-ray. It can, however, be treated another way and many people have responded well to that treatment. Whether I will be one of those remains to be seen. The treatment begins today.

I am telling you these facts because I want you to know the truth. I have always tried to be honest with you, and I can see no reason to change now. My days may be many; they may be not so many. Whatever the length of time may be, I shall live with one major purpose: to take the fear out of cancer. Thousands have been cured and are now living a normal life. Thousands have not been cured, but they have faced it without fear or dread. It helps just to be able to talk about it. Right now, the less said or written to me about it, the better.

You will help me most by accepting it quietly, trustfully; but not whispering about it; by expecting and hoping for the best; and then, by leaving the whole thing in the hands of Him Who alone sends us out and calls us in.

You and "the dear old Church" will always be in my mind and heart wherever I am, and whether I can do little or much. Whatever happens in the future, nothing can blot out my remembrance of how much the people of this Church have done for me in the last thirty years, how good they have been to me.

Sincerely, your friend and Rector,

# THE ADVANCED STAGE OF CANCER
# (STAGE 3)

THE advanced stage of cancer is reached when it is medically determined that the disease has spread to other parts of the body and that there is no way to stop further spread. Death is almost inevitable, although not necessarily quick. Medical procedures are available which may control ongoing growth but usually for a limited time. At least, they will lessen pain and discomfort.

The medical team, the patient and his family realize that the fears of the earlier stages of the disease have become a reality. They know that death is near, yet not usually imminent, and that they must endure together a period of waiting that is fraught with uncertainties. The doctor usually cannot estimate realistically how much time the patient has left. It depends on whether the various medical procedures have any effect on the rapidly growing disease. It is rare that a patient at this stage lives longer than one year. However, present-day use of relatively new drugs sometimes extends this period far beyond this.

The purpose of treatment at this stage is to try to slow up the ongoing disease process and at the same time to make the patient as comfortable as possible. For the doctor, paramedical personnel, patient, family and friends the task is to work out a comfortable rapport in which fear of dying and especially feelings of abandonment for all will be lessened. At this stage, feelings of rejection for the patient are often harder to bear than fear of death.

In fact, feelings of rejection reach their peak at this stage — feelings which can be dealt with, provided the caregivers are aware that this reaction usually is present, whether expressed or not. The burden falls most heavily on the person, usually a husband or wife, son or daughter, who has chief responsibility for care. Often this primary caregiver needs help.

The physician can offer support to the primary caregivers by assuring them that they are doing everything possible for the patient. But the physician should also be alert to the primary family caregiver's physical and emotional needs and be prepared to suggest and arrange professional counseling when it is needed. The primary caregiver inevitably becomes the most rejected individual in the total situation. His degree of rejection increases as the life of the patient is prolonged. Not only do the physician and paramedical personnel tend to shun him, but the patient himself frequently withdraws from those closest to him.

Denial and depression are the patient's dominant reactions as he becomes increasingly aware of his impending death. They are seemingly contradictory, but are in fact complementary coping devices which serve as a buffer against the painful shock of full realization. Once the primary caregiver is cognizant that the patient's new behavior pattern is not only normal but also a constructive way of managing, he can once again take his cues from the patient. The advanced cancer patient continues to provide the guidelines for effective support, which in turn affords personal satisfaction to the caregiver and greatly minimizes feelings of abandonment and rejection for all concerned.

The most difficult problem is to plan a future around an individual dying of cancer. There is much agreement that a patient who is sick enough to die knows it without being told.* One way that the medical team can ease their insecurity in caring for the patient is to make sure at this point especially that they make appropriate use of family members. This is the period to be aware of the fact that the family or one of its members is not only the patient's closest and most helpful caregiver in day and night care, but is also the medical team's closest ally.

Thus, the overriding goal is to help the patient live his remaining days with as much dignity and personal satisfaction as possible. This can be accomplished when he is given the right as far as possible to make his own decisions and to be part of the treatment team, and when the members of the health team including the patient's family are able to maintain their own equilibrium.

The advanced stage of cancer falls naturally into two periods:

---

*F. E. Adair, Cancer in our breast: interview with John Gunther. *Women's Home Companion,* February 1954.

the early stage covering "the time of telling" and "the time of waiting," and the late stage, "the time of dying." During all these periods there is an understandable frightened feeling. The grieving for what will be may need some type of counseling, depending on the course it takes and the symptoms it produces.

The medical team has many responsibilities and tasks during these two periods. There is much overlapping of roles among the physician, nurse, social workers and chaplain. Each one brings certain skills, but all have in common the task to offer emotional support. The doctor prescribes and carries out the medical therapy or therapies and offers interpretation and hope, the nurse provides nursing care with emotional support, the clinic social worker identifies resources for specific needs and is a trained counselor in the field of emotional support and the chaplain, representing a specific religious affiliation, has spiritual insights and knowledge. In addition, his training and experience in offering emotional support based on psychological concepts have been much developed in the past decade or two. All these representatives of the helping professions can offer support not only to the patients but to family members as well. Overlapping among them is good in the sense of increasing and sharing skills, but it does make it difficult to define the parameters of responsibility.

There are great similarities in the patient's physical abilities and behavioral patterns at these two periods. These require specific services. For all involved, knowledge of what to expect, what to do and where to go for help is of increasing importance.

The patterns I describe in this chapter have reappeared so frequently that they can be anticipated and used as guides. The Italian Roman Catholic housewife, the Jewish merchant, the black Baptist schoolteacher, the Greek Orthodox small business woman, the Lutheran factory worker, the Protestant bank president and the atheist philosopher — all appeared to choose similar coping methods to carry through with their responsibilities to others and to themselves.

## The Time of Telling

In no disease does the physician in charge carry as much burden as in advanced cancer. The many crises, real and imagined, that arise as the disease progresses can be eased and tolerated best when the patient and his family are secure in accepting the physician's responsibility for total care. The physician himself must not doubt his ability to handle the case. There can be no doubt that his management of each patient is the single most important factor in making care in the advanced stage an art as well as a science.

Often medical students, interns, residents, nurses, clinic social workers and even chaplains, regardless of their fields of specialization, have had no preparation for communicating with the advanced cancer patient, although more attention is now paid to this problem. For the doctor, the dying patient represents failure. His drive to study and practice medicine or to engage in medical research derives from a desire to help sick people by curing or arresting lethal processes of disease. His goal is to keep people from dying. Therefore, when he is unable to cure or arrest cancer he is confounded by feelings of professional inadequacy, whether justified or not, and by anxieties about death and dying that must be worked through if he is to give the fullest measure of care to his cancer patients.

From my observations of physicians who are successful in managing their advanced cancer patients I have concluded that the physician in charge of such a case is most helpful when he:

1. understands and accepts his own reaction to the disease and to dying and death,

2. uses his personal knowledge of each individual patient as a guide to talking with him about his illness, rather than saying what he would want to be told himself under similar circumstances,

3. lets the patient take the lead in asking questions, but responds with simple, clear statements,

4. avoids overexplanation, over-reassurance, unnecessary circumlocution and untruths,

5. tells the family as much as he can about the hoped-for and probable effects of treatment and, at the same time, prepares them for whatever effects of deterioration they can expect as the disease progresses,

6. makes appropriate referral to other professional caregivers such as psychiatrists, nurses, social workers, mental health counselors or chaplains within or outside the medical setting, and makes clear what can be expected from each,

7. and, perhaps most important, assures all involved that, no

matter what turn the illness may take, there is always something, another procedure or medication, that he can employ. He recognizes that implicit in this statement is his own commitment to stand by the patient and his family throughout the difficult time that lies ahead.

When the physician-in-charge has determined that the patient's condition has reached the irreversible stage, he arranges a face-to-face interview to discuss his findings and treatment. A relative or friend is included if the patient wishes.

How the doctor informs the patient of the gravity of his situation affects the degree of trust reposed in him. Generally speaking, there are five approaches doctors use to convey to their patients the change in their medical status.

1. The best approach, in my opinion, is to explain truthfully to the patient that the malignancy has spread and that the situation now is very grave. At the same time, the doctor emphasizes that there are medical procedures that may control or slow up the disease for an indefinite period. Taking his clues from the patient, the doctor will say only as much as he thinks the patient would like to hear and can face.

2. Another approach doctors use is never to use the word cancer but to couch their explanation in such a way that the patient becomes aware that his life is in jeopardy.

3. Some doctors believe it is their responsibility and the patient's right to know the whole truth about his prognosis. These physicians kindly but firmly state that the malignancy has spread to such an extent that present medical procedures cannot appreciably halt the fast-moving disease.

4. Other doctors treat their patients as they think they would wish to be treated themselves, failing to take into account the differences between their patients and themselves.

5. Finally, there are physicians whose policy is never to tell the patient the truth and who, therefore, imply unrealistic hope for the medical procedures they are recommending.

I think the first way is best because it reflects thoughtful concern on the part of the physician for the patient's ability to cope with his illness, and yet it is basically truthful and straightforward. On the other hand, it does not tell the patient more than he needs or wants to know at this point. The most important factor in the doctor's approach is truthfulness. The patient should always be told something, and what he is told must be truthful. The doctor strengthens his relationship with his patient when the patient feels that no matter what happens the doctor can be trusted to respond as honestly as the patient wishes.

Furthermore, the doctor should be aware of what the patient has found out about his condition. It is easy to underestimate or ignore how much the cancer patient already knows; he will seldom admit to the doctor at this time what he has learned or inferred from hospital personnel and others. The admitting nurse, the tumor clinic secretary, the social worker, other physicians, medical students, even other patients may have hinted at the truth.

I agree with the psychiatrist with whom I once worked, who stated that "to tell or not to tell is seldom an urgent question. Contrary to popular expectations, . . . patients soon are aware that something is amiss, and closest relatives and friends are poor actors. Ineffective treatments, persistent symptoms, and slippery excuses or reponses to questions reveal the true state of things long before the doctor and family get around to talking about the diagnosis and if necessary, death."*

On the other hand, telling a patient more than he needs to know or more than he can cope with can cause undue anxiety and threaten his ability to adjust to what lies ahead. It is a good philosophy that you need not tell the whole truth, but whatever you say must be truthful.

Occasionally, patients insist on knowing whether their situation has become "hopeless." In such cases, the doctor usually admits the seriousness of the patient's condition but returns as swiftly as is appropriate to how the proposed new treatment will slow up the disease process and at the same time relieve discomfort. The rare patient who does ask directly whether the disease is hopeless almost always does so for some specific reason. He wishes to change his will or make provision for a dependent person. I remember one case in which he wanted to be sure that his eyes would be donated to the eye bank.

The patient rarely is so direct again to his doctor, although he may remind one or more of his other caregivers of the specific task he

---

*A. D. Weisman, The patient with a fatal illness – to tell or not to tell. *JAMA.,* *196*:201, 646-648.

wishes to be taken care of. It is interesting that both the doctor and his patient seem to expect mutual evasiveness in this first confrontation with the known evidence of the spread of the patient's malignancy. The patient almost always accepts the new medical program even if he suspects the whole truth.

My studies have shown that no matter how the patient is told of his current life-threatening condition, he usually accepts his doctor with remarkable understanding and lack of criticism.

## Explaining the New Treatment Plan

Whatever way the doctor chooses to tell the patient about his altered medical status, he will emphasize that the purpose of the new treatment plan is to alleviate the symptoms and slow down the progress of the disease. He explains any change in procedure from previous treatment programs which may require a different specialist, a new method or a new setting, and makes clear whether he or another physician will be in charge. He will give the patient enough information about his condition so that treatment can proceed without hindrance.

There are many medical procedures that are available to make the patient as comfortable as possible. In choosing a treatment program, the doctor takes into consideration the patient's medical needs and his adjustment to his illness. He also thinks of the family's ability to care for the sick person.

Usually drugs to control or suppress the progress of the disease are administered, orally or by injection, at regular intervals in the doctor's office or at the clinic. X-ray treatment over a period of days or weeks also may be prescribed. Sometimes the patient's treatment program calls for both therapies concurrently.

Surgery to combat the progress of the disease is rarely done at this stage, primarily because the surgery might not prove helpful but also because the discomfort from an operation would only compound the patient's burden. However, neurological procedures for the relief of pain, such as nerve resection or cordotomy (the severance of sensory nerves) are sometimes carried out when medication cannot make the patient sufficiently comfortable. Most commonly, tranquilizers or sedatives such as codeine or Demerol® are adequate to relieve pain.

The patient's physician may also refer the patient to a

chemotherapist, neurologist, radiologist or psychiatrist for suggestions about different or new medications. The psychiatrist can suggest medications or supportive techniques that the physician can administer and supervise to relieve an angry, guilty or excessively frightened or depressed patient. In some instances, the psychiatrist may recommend direct psychotherapy as the optimum method of treating the patient's uncontrolled feelings.

The question of who should take responsibility for relieving the patient's anxiety was answered by a psychiatrist friend of mine. He said that although it would appear that the emotional and interpersonal aspects of advanced cancer should be within the province of the psychiatrist, this is frequently not the case. They must be dealt with in great measure, if not exclusively, by the attending physician. Often it frightens rather than helps the patient with advanced cancer to consider himself emotionally ill in addition to having a fatal illness. The psychiatrist's usefulness in these situations remains usually within the field of consultation.

The physician can offer help by arranging a face-to-face meeting in which he allows himself to be freer about his own thoughts of cancer. This is a good way to help the patient uncover or reveal the underlying reasons for his present behavior. This procedure may be continued by the appropriate caregiver selected by the physician. By this method, the patient retains confidence in his physician and the others who are caring for him, and in himself as well.

In my experience, individual psychotherapy for the advanced cancer patient, while rarely called for, has produced excellent results. And the patient should have access to this type of treatment if either he or his physician sees the need for it. One surgeon, discussing this question with me, said that a counselor might be included in the medical team when a patient, family member or friend displays excessive fear, anger, guilt or deep depression.

At this time, I am opposed to group therapy for advanced cancer patients for I believe that many need to mourn their condition by themselves or with their loved ones before they can cope with it in their own way.

In addition, I strongly feel that the periodic deaths of members of the group would be more than many patients could, or should, endure.

Recently I was asked my advice by a physician who was troubled by the depression he noted in a patient who had recently been operated on for a brain tumor. Following surgery the neurosurgeon had told the patient that the tumor was malignant. The physician asked me two questions: Did I think the patient should be seen by the psychiatrist? Did I think it would be helpful for her to have a visit from the other patient of his, similarly ill, who was adjusting well to her extensive cancer of the breast? When I reviewed the patient's former coping patterns it was my opinion that this particular woman, who had always been somewhat remote, needed time to withdraw and to think things through by herself before she could resume her former calm, restrained manner. Also, I thought it would be unwise to subject her to seeing another person in about the same stage of a malignancy whose reactions differed from hers.

The doctor followed my advice and found that I was right in my answers to both questions. After several days of almost complete silence, the patient's symptoms of depression lifted. Both she and her husband avoided seeing the acquaintance who was similarly ill.

The physician-in-charge may change as new medical procedures are tried or if the setting of medical care is shifted. Both the patient and his family will accept these changes as long as they are informed about who is responsible for the patient's total care. They must know who can be called in emergencies and who will make final decisions. The physician-in-charge may consult with other colleagues; he may refer the patient to another doctor for a specific type of examination, treatment or other service; he may ask another helping person, professional or nonprofessional, within or outside the setting, to assist him in supporting the patient and his family. However, he remains the leader of the medical team.

In other words, as the leader of the medical team the physician-in-charge attempts to maintain an active relationship with the patient and his family, particularly the most involved family caregiver. He shares with the other caregivers pertinent information relative to the patient's medical situation: the patient's understanding of his prognosis, his reactions to what he has been told and the current plans for management of his medical and personal needs and wishes.

The physician especially can support the advanced cancer patient by visiting at regular and expected intervals, or by clearly designating an associate or assistant who will alternate with him in the medical treatment and care. The patient is greatly relieved if he knows at the end of each visit when the doctor will return. If the physician is going away briefly or for a long period it is well to share this information with the patient and the family.

In particular, the physician who has confronted and accepted his own fears about death and dying possesses an important component of self-awareness and composure that should enable him to effectively manage encounters with patients facing extinction of life.

### How the Patient Reacts

The patient in the early advanced stage, even prior to his talk with the doctor, usually knows or suspects that his condition is deteriorating, is probably hopeless and will end in death. He wonders when, how and even why. But in confrontation with his physician he seldom voices these disturbing questions — questions he realizes are equally disturbing to the doctor. He anticipates the likelihood that the doctor will avoid as much as he can any talk about the fact that the disease is irreversible. He understands and is almost prepared for the doctor's dilemma and disappointment. Perhaps he is even relieved that he and the doctor do not have to spell out the whole truth of the changed situation.

The patient and his physician concentrate now on treatment. The patient may ask who will administer the medical procedure, how often and where he should go to get it, and he certainly will ask who his doctor will be during treatments. He agrees that the physician cannot give all the answers, that they will both have to wait and see how effective a particular drug may or may not be.

Without actually communicating as they did in the earlier stages of the disease when the partnership was free of subterfuge and evasion, the doctor and his patient now resume a kind of partnership where the most important things are left unsaid but are understood by both parties.

This does not mar the doctor-patient relationship. I have rarely known a patient in the advanced stage to leave his doctor for anything that the latter has left unsaid or for anything said in an unsympathetic or brusque manner, or even for ignoring the patient's particularly troubling questions. I remember the doctor who said to me, "When a patient asks me a question I don't want to answer, I change the subject as quickly as I can and find an excuse to leave the room." The patients of this doctor never asked for a replacement and always gave him a friendly greeting and a thank-you at the end.

What becomes most apparent is the fact that the patient says as little as possible to his doctor at the time he is told. More frequently than one might suppose, he leaves the doctor's office without expressing any of his fears. The doctor's willingness to keep on trying new treatment methods reassures him of his continuing concern. As one doctor says, "There is always something else I can try." The byline "we'll have to wait and see" brings a satisfactory ending to this excruciatingly difficult talk.

## What the Doctor Tells the Family

The doctor's interview with the family usually takes place in the patient's absence. Whatever information he may have given the patient, the doctor tells the family, or at least one member or close friend, the full significance of his findings. He will state frankly that because the malignancy may no longer be controlled for any appreciable length of time, the patient will almost certainly not survive. He outlines the medical procedures that he has chosen, or states that he will consult with others before making final plans regarding further medical procedures. The goal now is to try to slow the disease and relieve pain.

The family in most instances respond by accepting the doctor's treatment plan and committing themselves to help in whatever way they can. However. the shock and disappointment of hearing that there is little realistic hope for lengthening the life span indefinitely give rise to many troubling questions. One of the first questions is whether the patient knows that his condition is probably hopeless. The family members are afraid that they may unwittingly do or say something that will reveal the truth. Worse, they are afraid of breaking down in front of him.

The doctor should let the family know what he has told the patient. He should also mention, as has been pointed out, that a patient who is gravely ill usually knows the truth anyway. The doctor can also reassure the family that a display of emotion, far from being harmful, shows the sick person how much he is loved. But he does suggest that discussions of diagnosis and outlook should take place only if and when the patient himself wishes to bring up the subject. Family members should not tell the patient what they would want to hear; rather, they should listen carefully to what the patient asks directly or appears to want to know.

In addition, the doctor may advise that those in the family group who do not know the truth should be told. Even children should have some knowledge of the patient's true situation. Individual family members, including children, may need to talk to a trusted friend or perhaps a member of the medical team, such as a physician, a nurse, clinic social worker or chaplain or family member about their own reactions and relationship with the patient and the feelings of sadness which now disturb them. Understanding something about the seriousness of the patient's condition will also help them to understand his behavior and then to act appropriately. On the other hand, a "hush-hush" atmosphere where no one admits how ill the patient really is fools no one, and in the long run intensifies the distress of the patient, his family and close friends.

The family wonders what physical and emotional changes the patient will undergo, how and where he will die, what will be their responsibility in his care. Will they be able to carry on the household or financial burdens of the patient during his illness and after he is gone? The patient has questions too, but the family is more open than the patient about asking. The doctor should encourage them, as he did the patient, to reveal their anxieties. His continuing interest in them throughout the patient's illness can be an invaluable source of strength. He should emphasize that if he is unavailable, there are others on the medical team, such as a particular nurse or social worker, who can help. Also at this period the doctor has an impression of how much communication the family will want or will impose on him. A physician may be relieved of a constant questioning or difficult family member by introducing a team member, a social worker or chaplain to act as his helper in such a situation.

## Emergence of the Primary Family Caregiver

As the physician makes his report to the assembled family members, he will note their varying responses and perhaps make sure that everyone fully understands what he has heard. He will usually be able to discern from the reactions of those present which one of them will become the primary family caregiver, someone emotionally close to the patient. This is the one who will bear the main burden of the patient's illness and dying. He will be called upon to provide most of the patient's physical care at home and emotional support. He is the physician's closest ally, and for this reason he should be able to turn to the doctor or someone the doctor designates, such as the nurse, chaplain or social worker, for compounding the chief family caregiver's deep concern for the patient is his own nagging doubt about his ability to withstand the impending pressures.

The doctor should tell this person in charge just what will happen to the patient, as well as he can predict, and what the caregiver should be prepared to do for him. By taking the time to explain these matters, the doctor demonstrates his respect for his most important ally and reassures him that he will stand by to help.

## The Responsibility of the Caregivers

The fact that treatment in some instances does have good results may give the patient hope that his condition will continue to improve. If the caregivers can anticipate and understand the patient's medical and emotional ups and downs, as well as their own reactions to cancer and dying and death, they can provide better care.

I do not wish to imply that each caregiver needs to undergo some form of psychotherapy in order to understand his own reactions. However, if a caregiver considers that nothing helpful can be done for the patient, or that a prescribed treatment is unacceptable, repellent or unavailing, or that the cancer site is repugnant, he should consult with the physician or a counselor to help him sort out his thoughts and decide whether or how much he should participate in the patient's care. Too frequently, the nurse, social worker, laboratory technician, even the minister and physician, shield themselves from the problems presented by caring for an advanced cancer patient. Instead of confronting the issues, they remain silent, quickly withdraw or refer all questions to a higher authority.

A young nurse caring for a patient with advanced carcinoma of the breast later confessed,

> Every day when I entered her room, I felt a strong upsurge of feelings of guilt. I was going to live while she of my own age was about to die. I knew she wanted to talk to me, but I always turned it into something light, a little joke, or into some evasive reassurance which had to fail. The patient knew and I knew. But as she saw my desperate attempt to escape and felt my anxiety, she took pity on me and kept to herself what she wanted to share with another human being — and so she died and did not bother me.*

Today most patients are sophisticated about medical matters; it is no longer possible to sustain a fictional prognosis over a lengthy period of illness. The patients know that the caregivers have at least some of the answers, so that to continually sidestep issues the patient may raise can only increase his emotional stress. All the caregivers can help by adopting an open attitude. They should be able to show the patient that there is nothing about his illness, the effect of treatment or his reactions to the present crisis which cannot be understood and dealt with.

A 32-year-old psychologist talked about her husband's life during the waiting period. She said he

> never verbalized thoughts of death, but his unconscious behavior always indicated that he knew he was going to die soon. He had already taken care of the things a mature man would do. He had made sure that our financial house was in order. He certainly did not give me any profound lecture about what I should do now or later. We had sort of a quiet understanding . . .

---

*I. S. Wolfe, The magnificence of understanding. In *Should the Patient Know the Truth?* ed. by Samuel Standard and Helmut Nathan (New York, Springer Publishing Co., 1955), p. 32.

When he would seem extremely depressed, making a remark that he was maybe "a dead man," my response usually was, "What can I say to comfort you?" I never denied the fact or confirmed that he undoubtedly was going to die soon. I felt that this was something that did not have to be denied or confirmed.

Probably the hardest task of any of the advanced cancer patient's caregivers is to bear silences or, when necessary, to confine conversation to remarks that attempt to be supportive while at the same time offering comfort. There is no escape from fundamental loneliness; however, awareness of what is happening to the patient and what to expect from him can sustain his dignity and allow him to feel that he remains in control of himself and the circumstances of his life.

If the caregivers can understand this, then they will be able to go on caring for the patient without excessive anxiety or self-reproach. Understanding the patient's moods also embodies recognition of his right to stipulate the degree of intimacy with others that he can bear, that right which I hold most important for him to effectively cope with his illness. Everything the patient says, implies or actually does leaves no doubt that it is he alone who takes the lead in releasing those who care for him, especially the physician, family and friends, from any obligation to share mutual anxieties.

## *Primary Family Caregiver's Special Role*

The primary family caregiver, usually the wife, mother, daughter or possibly the husband of the patient if he is no longer employed outside the home, but always someone on whom the patient has depended deeply in the past, undertakes many tasks in caring for the patient.

In my experience, she accepts her role without question and enters into this most painful task without complaint. From the start, she functions as a source of strength and care combining many roles, any one of which would in other circumstances be considered a major responsibility in itself. She must be all of the following, usually with no previous experience and little if any professional direction: (1) the homemaker, planning the patient's activities and medical regimen and providing the essentials of daily living; (2) the nurse's aide, administering the at-home medical procedures; (3) the protector, who monitors the contacts of others with the patient; (4) the counselor, who supports the patient's acknowledged fears and accepts the patient's defenses of denial and symptoms of depression.

The primary family caregiver has a difficult emotional task. She must sustain the patient's emotional and physical status while preparing for her own forthcoming bereavement. Both she and the patient are beset by strong fears of death and dying, and of abandonment by the physician in particular. Yet, the primary family caregiver and the patient both decide to cope with their fears without revealing them, to avoid upsetting each other and to maintain an acceptable image of themselves.

The doctor can emphasize the importance of the primary family caregiver's role by letting her know that he depends on her to see that his recommendations for care are followed. The primary family caregiver responds by feeling both satisfaction and a greater sense of identity when her responsibility is pointed out. The doctor can also tactfully let the other family members know that their support of the primary family caregiver can help to ease her burden.

The primary family caregiver, so closely bound to the hopelessly ill patient by emotional need and the necessity of day and night care, often has the most to lose by the patient's death. Of all those involved, she should receive attention to help in planning not only for the patient's care, but also for her own adjustment after the patient's death. Years of attempting to resolve anger, guilt and other emotional disturbances lingering in persons who cared for dying loved ones without such help have convinced me that this matter is fully as important as assuring optimal physical and emotional support for the patient.

By repressing and concealing her feelings during the time of the patient's illness and death, the primary family caregiver may leave unresolved many areas of conflict in her relationship with the patient that can cripple her ability to offer her optimum support and to cope with life after loss.

## The Counselor as a Member of the Medical Team

When the physician-in-charge is planning the patient's medical program, he would do well to include a counselor for the patient or his family. This will probably be a professional helper — a nurse, social worker or clergyman. This person should be identified as a member of the medical team at the outset of treatment. If she is a nurse or social worker, she will be available to the patient and his family for ongoing help. She can be of immeasurable help to the doctor to clarify the patient's medical status and, more important, to help him recognize why the patient may be reacting in a baffling way. She can suggest how these uncomfortable feelings can be lessened or eradicated. And this same counselor can be available whether the patient remains at home, travels at stated intervals to the clinic or resides in a nursing home or chronic hospital. The family can readily reach her when a specific service is needed or an emotional crisis occurs.

I remember a patient, a schoolteacher of forty, who was about to be discharged to her own home. She and her husband seemed a devoted couple. Through community resources, which included a visiting nurse, a homemaker, a Red Cross volunteer and emergency care by a local physician, I had made sure that she would have the services needed for her care at home and for the weekly visits to the hospital. However, on the very morning she was to leave the hospital I received a call. The patient had something she had to tell me. With curtains drawn, and whispering, she told me she was afraid to go home. She was ashamed to tell the doctor that her husband was an alcoholic who frequently abused her. A change in plan was made immediately, and the woman was transferred to a nursing home for the remainder of her life. The doctor explained to both of them that her medical and nursing needs had become far too great for her to be taken care of at home.

In this case, the patient found it easier to talk to me than to her doctor, who represented an authority figure. In my private practice I have found that patients and their families frequently find it easier to bring their nonmedical concerns to me than to the physician, whom they hesitate to bother. Being available to them by telephone at my office and home gives them the confidence of my continued interest, and when they come in to see me I have the time to listen and to counsel. Often I serve as the bridge between the doctor and the patient's family, helping to clarify questions which the family has been unwilling to discuss with the busy physician.

Religious faith comforts and supports many patients and should be considered in any program for optimum management, especially in the terminal stage. Regular visits by the chaplain are especially effective when the medical personnel and clergyman are partners in treatment. Problems arise when a particular physician abdicates his services upon learning of the chaplain's visits.

I remember the 31-year-old chemist who was dying of cancer of the rectum. After a weekend away from the hospital, I went to see him in the ward. His greeting was, "I thought you, too, had deserted me!" I questioned him and found that his physician, a young man of similar age, had not visited him for the past five days. The Protestant chaplain was now making the only daily visits. The patient was eager to see his doctor and felt excessively hostile and bitter that now when he needed him most he no longer made daily visits.

Later in the day I questioned the particular doctor, who was a Catholic. He said, "If I was as sick as that young man I would want my priest. He is a Protestant, although I guess a nonpracticing one, so I thought the time had come for his care to be in the hands of a spiritual counselor rather than a medical practitioner." It did not take much explanation on my part to assure this usually sensitive young physician that, although the clergyman was of help, the patient still needed his doctor more than ever to care for and comfort him until the end. This also is an example of overidentification of one young scientist to another.

## The Time of Waiting

After the doctor tells the patient and his family about the revised diagnosis and prognosis, the time of waiting begins, a time that everyone realizes will undoubtedly end with the death of the patient. The patient and those who care for him alternate relentlessly between unrealistic upsurges of hope, usually prompted by a good response to a particular medication or treatment procedure, and episodes of deep despair, when the truth of the patient's condition cannot be denied. The strain of knowing that the patient will die, while he continues to live, creates major emotional stresses. Both the sick person and his caregivers want his life to be prolonged, yet at the same time and for many reasons they often wish the end to come soon.

During the early advanced stage, the cancer patient may be wholly or partially ambulatory, able to care for himself and to travel, perhaps even drive himself to a clinic or a physician's office for medical treatment. Specific medical procedures such as changing dressings or colostomy irrigations may be carried out by the patient himself or by a family member trained by a visiting nurse or in the hospital prior to the patient's discharge. The services of a visiting nurse are recommended by the physician-in-charge and carried out by the nurse or social worker.

One of the most difficult problems for the patient at this time is the change in life style. While he does not need the presence or constant attention of someone else in the home, nor has he yet become a physical burden to his family, he usually can no longer work on a full-time basis. He can, however, carry on with the activities of daily living, pursue hobbies of a sedentary nature and take part in some social activities. He may work part time, especially if he is self-employed or in a profession that permits working hours to be conveniently adjusted. If the patient's income is insufficient, a social worker at the hospital or in the community may arrange financial assistance. If the patient is a housewife, she must be relieved of some of her tasks either by a family member, friend or a homemaker. The services of a homemaker can be arranged through community and private social agencies.

The need for financial aid constitutes an added emotional burden for the patient and his family. The social worker or some other counselor should explain that the funds that make private or public assistance possible are contributed by all members of society, including the patient himself, and that the patient has a socially acceptable right to such funds. By explaining the matter in this way and giving the patient and his family the opportunity to communicate their feelings about aid from private or public sources, the counselor can help them accept this needed support.

It is unwise for an advanced cancer patient to consider moving from his home in an effort to reduce living costs, except in extreme circumstances of physical or financial need. Taking the patient out of his familiar environment means one more stressful change he must accept. Most patients can adapt to their altered life styles if circumstances are at all favorable.

Transportation for visits to the doctor may have to be arranged, but usually family members and friends are quick to be helpful once they are told something about the situation. Often the patient wants to continue to drive, particularly to see his doctor.

To help preserve his self-image and his will to go on living, the patient should be encouraged to be as independent and physically active as he can and wishes to be. When his activities need to be curtailed, the reason should be explained to friends, employers or others who are involved. Unlike diseases such as heart disease, cancer is not worsened by physical activity. Becoming overtired or overanxious does not affect the spread of this particular disease, and there is little chance of a sudden or acute attack. For these reasons, a cancer patient's activities, even if they are excessive, need not cause alarm to his family and friends.

### The Patient's Emotional Response

I have found denial and depression to be the most disturbing reactions during this time of waiting.* Depression, though it may alarm the caregivers by its apparent severity, may permit the patient to adjust to his poor prognosis. He goes through a kind of mourning perhaps for the person he has been, perhaps for the person that he will never be. It may also be a way of "catching up" to what is happening to him, adjusting to life as a person who knows he will die in the foreseeable future. This period of mourning often takes the form of weeping spells which may add to the discomfort and sorrow of those around him. Yet these evidences of understandable depression should be allowed. A patient of mine, Adele B., recently told me that the nurses in the

---

*R. D. Abrams, Denial and depression in the terminal cancer patient — a clue for management. *Psychiatr Q, 45*:394-404, November 3, 1971.

hospital practically insisted that she take a tranquilizer to stop her weeping. Adele refused. She said she needed to cry and knew it would make her feel better.

As soon as the new treatment starts, however, the symptoms of depression ease and alternate with symptoms of denial. The two can even occur simultaneously. The alternation of the patient's moods is upsetting to the caregiver, who finds it difficult to know how to respond appropriately. The caregiver is aware that the patient may say or imply at the same meeting both that he will die and that he will live. No wonder the caregiver is perplexed about which state of mind — hope or despair — the patient wants him to respond to. This results in a dilemma which usually can be ameliorated by saying nothing, yet indicating by nonverbal methods concern for his fear of death and acceptance of his hope of living.

For the patient, denial and depression enable him to turn his feelings inward and withdraw from intimate communication. Denial permits him to avoid direct confrontation with the grave significance of his present deteriorating condition and symptoms of depression, and helps him to keep from expressing any unpleasant, angry or fearful feelings from which he may be suffering. He fears that any angry or fearful outbursts, especially to his doctor, would mar the self-image he so desperately wishes to maintain.

These behavioral devices of denial and depression broadly affect the advanced cancer patient's relationships with his caregivers and family. At this waiting period, the patient's retreat from formerly close relationships, hinted at in the advancing stage, becomes the dominant factor in his coping with his illness. He may see his friends, but he does not communicate his anxieties to them. It is important for the friends to understand that this is the usual reaction and does not mean they have said something hurting.

The contact with friends may be relatively superficial when they meet, but the need for it is real. This was expressed by a middle-aged woman with lung cancer who wrote on her Christmas card to a few friends, "Come soon, don't wait too long." The patient may let his friends know about his present condition, but when face-to-face with them he talks about his disabilities or the effect of medication, but not about the disease. A physician with terminal cancer, for example, told me that his spasms of pain were caused "by my ticker, not that other thing."

The more I have seen patients in the early advanced stage, the more I have been surprised at the intensity of their activities, mental and physical. Yet the extreme physical activity may change for no reason from independence to a desire to lean on others. "You decide for me," the patient will say in one breath and in the next he will be furious, especially at those closest to him, for not permitting him to make all his own decisions — to drive his car, do some work, participate in social gatherings or make plans for trips he knows he will never be able to make.

He may be compulsive about whatever he is doing, even to the extent of shutting out what is going on around him. I recall that the same physician who insisted it was his heart that was his main trouble kept the record player blasting away and even attempted to sing along with his favorite operatic records to blot out any conversation which might intrude on his denial. Often he was compulsively engaged in writing at his desk. The combination of the record player distraction and the preoccupation with professional responsibilities afforded him a method of withdrawal which became a burden to friends and family alike.

Whatever form his activity may take, the patient appears to want to avoid at all costs embarrassing or emotional scenes. For each visit to his doctor, he often prepares a list of questions about his symptoms, but almost never about the disease process itself. He never disturbs the doctor between visits unless absolutely necessary. If the doctor must be reached, the patient insists on making the call himself. He is determined to remain responsible for all decisions that affect himself as long as possible.

Many patients even take the responsibility for remaining at home, or being taken care of at some appropriate facility. They indicate with great insight where and by whom care should be provided. The caregivers, by giving the patients an opportunity to make their own plans, reinforce their inclusion in the treatment team. Most patients at this stage want to remain at home.

However, there are exceptions. One was Raphael, the 19-year-old whose case I discussed in Chapter 2. He had previously lived in harmony with his mother. (He was the youngest of five children and his mother's favorite.) When his disease became irreversible, he was discharged to his home, with bimonthly clinic appointments. However, as time went on he became restive; finally, he suggested to his local family physician that it would be better for both him and his mother if he could be transferred to a nearby chronic cancer hospital. He explained that the anxiety and tension that both he and his mother were suffering were undermining their relationship. As the social worker on the case, I was asked to arrange the transfer. The new arrangement proved to be beneficial for both mother and son, as I was able to confirm in my weekly visits to the son and in my continued contact with his mother.

Many doctors wonder, especially when patients have not been told directly about the seriousness of their illness, whether their patients will make a will. I have found that regardless of other circumstances, the patient who has been responsible previously will put his house in order at this time as well. In fact, he feels driven to do so, whether he discusses it with anyone else or not. Usually, rather surreptitiously, the patient sees his lawyer about his will and perhaps leaves instructions to be read by his family after he is gone.

Another striking characteristic of the advanced cancer patient is that he resumes activities that he enjoyed in his early life. A 55-year-old carpenter, for example, took great pleasure in going to the beach every Sunday as he had done as a child, and began to go regularly to Friday night services at a nearby synagogue which he had not attended for years.

The patient is extremely concerned about leaving behind a good image of himself and wants his good deeds to be remembered. I recall a 40-year-old architect who took obvious satisfaction in the realization that the school buildings he had designed would serve as his memorial, especially for his children. Often the sick person will work compulsively to finish a book, or household renovation or some particular job.

The patient may also wonder about the effectiveness of his own or a colleague's life work. A psychiatrist, in the early advanced stage of cancer of the stomach, discussed with me his surgeon's inability to communicate with him at the time of his surgery. "Can we do away with these defenses?" he said more to himself than to me. "That is what the psychiatrists should be working on, instead of all this nonsense." I think he was questioning his ability to cope with his own crisis as well as pointing out new areas for study.

Some patients will discuss their impending death with their doctor, especially if they wish a specific plan to be carried out after death. For example, one patient wanted to be sure that his organs would be willed to the hospital where he had received treatment. But once the particular plan is established, it is seldom if ever referred to again.

Further evidence of the reluctance of these patients to talk in sensitive areas was noted when I was asked to obtain the cooperation of patients for staff psychiatrists interested in cancer patients' reactions to dying and death. All the patients reacted negatively to this suggestion (as did over 96 percent in another study in a distant medical center).* They remarked, "I don't feel equal to it," "I'm frightened by it," "I don't feel smart enough" or "It will remind me of the depressing things about my condition." Several patients stated frankly that they did not see how talking with a psychiatrist could possibly help others because "everyone is different." Yet these same patients were following unquestioningly a medical regimen they knew was also in the research phase.

Occasionally, a doctor will feel the need "to get the record straight" by sharing the truth with the patient. One doctor says he tells the truth "across the board" to all his cancer patients. In such a situation, the patient, because of his great dependence on his doctor, is like a member of a captive audience; he cannot leave the scene, even though he may wish to escape. He feels, however unreasonably, that he has to choose between being approved of or being abandoned, and he can only choose the former. While it may be painful for him, he usually will comply with the doctor's wish to discuss his prognosis. My observations concur with the recent findings of Dr. Hoyle Leigh, who, drawing on his experience as

*Chicago Tumor Institute Report, 1963 (unpublished).

psychiatric liaison on a neoplastic inpatient service, said that the majority of patients at this stage do not appear to need to communicate with their physicians about dying in order to cope with their hopeless condition.*

Many patients at times will talk about projected family, social or professional activities in which they know they will not be able to take part. They speak of meetings they will attend, reunions with family members and visits to faraway lands. At other times a patient will become angry and insist on knowing the truth. Later in the same day he may turn unbelievably benign. He may carry physical activity to a ritualistic pattern, then suddenly turn dependent and weak. These ambivalences are characteristic of the advanced stage.

When depressive remarks are made, they are almost always directed to the primary family caregiver, not to other members of the family or to friends, and practically never to the physician-in-charge. Aside from rare bitter outbursts, such references to dying and death take the form of statements, even joking remarks, rather than questions requiring answers. Patients may indicate preferences for funeral or burial arrangements. They may suggest that their mates remarry after they are gone, and even recommend a successor!

The caregivers usually find it difficult to respond when patients vent their underlying feelings of humiliation, frustration and rejection. "A year ago, when I was first admitted for surgery, I entered the hospital prepared to die, but following surgery I was resigned to live." "The doctors have not visited me for days, probably because they know there is nothing that they can do for me." "I've been around here for days and all I'm getting is the runaround."

There are instances, although they are relatively rare, when an advanced cancer patient is unable to cope with his anxieties. He may exhibit a frighteningly depressive state with excessive irritability, overt hostility, paranoia and threats of suicide. In my clinical experience, however, I know of no death of a cancer patient by suicide. This fact coincides with findings of other studies which

---

*Hoyle Leigh, Psychiatric liaison on a neoplastic in-patient service. Psychiatry in Medicine, 4:147-154, Spring, 1973.

indicate that it is only very rarely that a patient with cancer at any stage actually causes his own death.*

When a terminal patient is thus crying for help, interventive techniques must be considered. One physician who handled the situation with great sensitivity wrote, "When my middle son was dying of certain incurable complications I saw him become hostile and distrustful of everybody he loved best. It was making his final months dreadful for him and for us as well, until I came to him and spelled out every last word of the truth. We cried together, and from that time on he was close to us again, and we to him."

## The Doctor-Patient Relationship

As the disease progresses, the patient develops a growing dependence on his doctor. He thinks unconsciously that perhaps there will be a miracle, and, if so, clearly the doctor is the one who can make it happen. As the patient binds the doctor more closely to himself, he excludes everyone else from contact with the doctor. He insists on talking to the doctor himself, he drives himself to the clinic for treatment as long as he is able and if he permits his family to accompany him, he insists that they wait outside the treatment room.

Thus a psychological cleavage develops, with the patient and the doctor on one side and the family on the other. Essentially, the patient is withdrawing defensively from overt dependence on his family, which has now become too painful for all of them, and reposing his need for dependence on his doctor, where he can be safe from emotional repercussions. This seeming rejection of the family by the doctor and the patient adds to the family's distress. They should be helped to understand that the patient's withdrawal from them is not rejection (to which they need to respond defensively) but a protective device.

## The Primary Caregiver

Finally, there is need for a plan which takes into consideration

---

*A.D. Weisman, *On Dying and Denying.* New York, Behavioral Publications, 1973

preventive mental health procedures for the primary family caregiver. This has been proven by the verbatim data collected from the *Conjugal Bereavement Study,* Laboratory of Community Psychiatry, Harvard Medical School and also from data currently in my private practice. There is sufficient evidence from these two sources to confirm the recent findings of other investigators here and abroad that men and women under the age of forty-five who have lost a spouse develop a higher incidence of medical and mental ill health than the average population.* In the *Conjugal Bereavement Study,* 26 out of the total of 69 subjects died of cancer. In other words, these were not sudden or unexpected deaths. There was time to prepare.

But, at thirteen months after the loss, more than one half of these widows and widowers were found to have made a relatively "poor" adjustment. Only four of the 26 survivors had made themselves known or been referred to a hospital or community social worker during the spouse's illness, and only one of this group had had regular supportive therapy – this in spite of the fact that the place of treatment and death was in general hospitals and within communities with well-established and available social service or mental health facilities. Furthermore, there was no indication that ongoing support was sought from other professional individuals within or outside the medical setting, such as physicians, nurses, community health workers or chaplains.† Arranging for the family caregiver to get a day off each week is a simple yet important task which could be accomplished.

The *Conjugal Bereavement Study* corroborates a finding noted repeatedly by me and others in hospital settings, namely, that following the patient's death the primary family caregiver rarely returns for help to the setting where the patient was cared for. I used to think that to return to the scene of the tragedy was more than the survivor could bear. However, as a result of further study, it is now my impression that the primary family caregiver does not seek help because she no longer considers that she is significant.

---

*I. Glick, R. Weiss, and C. Murray Parkes, *The First Year of Bereavement.* New York, Wiley and Sons.

†R. D. Abrams, and M. Hindley, Bereavement in cancer – adjustment processes of surviving spouses under age 45. (In preparation).

The social worker and/or the chaplain can be of particular help to the family at this time by showing that they are available and that their help will be ongoing. The family caregiver who is referred by the observant physician can be helped to cope with the final separation.

## A Guide for Caregivers

In the management of patients during the waiting period, the following questions may be guides for the medical team and the most involved family members.

First, are the patient's devices of denial and depression helping him to maintain his life style or the image of himself that he can tolerate? Is he having more discomfort with feelings of inaccessibility, guilt or rejection than he can bear? Perhaps it is the caregiver who cannot tolerate the patient's seeming breakdown in logical thinking. Is the caregiver overwhelmed by feelings of inadequacy, guilt and rejection? Or is he becoming hostile, depressed and unable to get along with the patient as he now has become? The question is, "Who is adjusting adequately, the patient or the caregiver?"

If the patient is comfortable, then it would appear that his wishes for the management of his situation, as implied in the clues he usually provides, should be respected and maintained. This should be the caregiver's goal. If the caregiver is so disturbed that he can no longer help and is now avoiding the patient, then it would appear that he should be made aware of his inappropriate involvement. He should understand his own reactions. Insight into one's own attitude about dying makes it possible to chart the course which will be most helpful in each situation.

I find that denial and depression are the significant reactions that affect the roles of the caregivers. When these reactions appear to signify a change in the patient's logical thinking, they cause a gap between the patient and his caregivers. The caregivers must accept the fact that now the patient is different. These maneuvers are the paths he selects to maintain an acceptable image of himself and to insure the kind of legacy he wishes to leave behind. Intervention should be considered only when the patient displays behavior that the patient, not the caregiver, cannot tolerate.

CHAPTER 4

# THE LATE ADVANCED STAGE
# (STAGE 3)

$A$ CANCER patient is considered to be in the late advanced stage, the terminal period, when extension of the disease has spread to vital organs or when all therapy has become ineffectual. The patient frequently shows an emotional detachment from life (medically known as decathexis) and has reached the point where he does not have the strength or will to do things for himself. Further treatment is palliative only. Acute episodes of illness with uncontrollable pain, diarrhea and excessive fear or symptoms of depression may occur between the insidious onset of this condition and death. Hospitalization may or may not be needed. This period may last only a few hours or days, or it may last several weeks, rarely months.

When the time of dying is reached, the agitation that marked the patient's behavior during the early advanced stage is replaced by a calm, suspended hopelessness, expressed as wordless resignation. The family members react to the news that the patient has entered the final medical crisis with great sorrow, but also with some feeling of relief — although seldom expressed — that the end of the ordeal is at hand.

While the final outcome of this medical crisis is irrevocable, there are means by which all who care for the patient can meet his needs and their own satisfactorily. Perhaps most important for all caregivers to know is the fact that silence is the language of this period, as exemplified by the patient's withdrawal and regression to a state of almost total dependency. But nonverbal communication that transmits understanding and even sorrow is not only acceptable but important to the patient's need for dependency, regression and resignation. This chapter will consider how the patient's caregivers can best use this knowledge to support the patient as he wishes to be supported and thereby derive satisfaction from their care of him.

## Medication

Many forms of palliation through sedation are available to relieve the patient's suffering, both emotional and physical, at this time. Tranquilizers, codeine, Demerol and morphine are most commonly used. Recently lysergic acid (LSD) has been used experimentally in some terminal cancer patients, but only after the other drugs had become ineffective. Good responses were noted most often when this medication was combined with psychotherapy.* In England, heroin has been given trials in these patients with good results, since heroin does not dull the senses as morphine does when dosages are increased.† However, in this country heroin is not legally available for any medical purpose.

The doctor naturally has the authority in this issue, but the patient can be consulted profitably regarding his medication. He may, for example, be willing to endure some pain in order to remain clear-headed during this final period, or he may prefer a strong dose of pain-killing medication that will also make him sleepy and less mentally alert. In either case, the patient and his family should be informed of the effects the suggested drugs will have, both positive and negative.

Usually the patient is almost completely bedridden and unable to take care of even the most elementary of his physical needs. Depending on the kind and amount of medication he is receiving, he may have difficulty staying awake for more than short periods at a time. His mind usually is clear, but he specifically avoids making decisions that require concentration. He wants to be taken care of, as indeed he should be. As a dying department store executive muttered, almost to himself, when told that a colleague

---

*I. S. Groff, W. N. Pahnke, L. E. Goodman, and A. A. Kurland, LSD: Psychedelic drug-assisted psychotherapy in patients with terminal cancer, Part 2. *JAMA, 212*:1856, 1970.

†Cecily Saunders, The treatment of intractable pain in terminal cancer. *Proc R Soc Med, 56(3)*:195-197, 1963.

requested him to make a policy decision, "He'd better decide himself — he'll have to soon enough."

## Problems of Home Care

Planning for the patient's care at home in the final stage of his illness can be complicated by his specific needs, as illustrated in the following letter to me from a 32-year-old woman discharged to her home after extensive surgery for carcinoma of the cervix.

I wonder if you'd mind if I appealed to your good nature once again? We have been trying to manage without asking for further help from you, but we are just getting deeper in debt, with one creditor now threatening attachment of pay.

It costs us on the average of $30.00 a week for my supplies: unsterile cotton, cellucotton and cheese cloth, not counting the small things such as Kleenex,® aspirin, adhesive, Vaseline,® etc. This, together with the food, insurance, oil and laundry, eats up a week's pay in no time, leaving nothing for the ordinary bills like gas, electricity, telephone, etc., of which we pay half. Then there are shoes, socks and so on, for my oldest boy.

My husband called my druggist, but they quote retail prices and they said they couldn't quote the hospital prices, except by the truckload.

Do you think it would do any good to ask the Red Cross for help, and if so how would I go about it? If we could manage to get some of the things paid for, it sure would mean a lot.

Also, when asking about lap pads, what other name do they go by? What we do now is make the pads ourselves, and it's pretty monotonous at times, especially if I don't feel too good.

I am coming along slow but sure, I hope. I have my good days and I have my bad ones, and sometimes I have pretty mean nights, but I'll try to make the best of things for three months, as they would like to have me do. I called on the 17th and wanted to talk to Dr. M. [intern] or Dr. T. [resident], but of course the doctors are changed around again, so maybe if you think of it sometime when you are talking to Dr. M. or Dr. P. [surgical chief], you would tell them my right foot and leg are swelling again all the time, so when I'm up I keep it bandaged. Would an elastic stocking be more successful? Yesterday my right foot and ankle were also swollen and my leg is kind of stiff feeling.

The doctor I spoke to in MGH Group Service said to take

Nembutal® as a sleeping pill, which I've been doing, but it isn't always successful. I have taken phenobarbitol and also Luminal,® the latter having helped a little more. I'd like to know more about taking these, too. Also, when I was in there on June 5th, Dr. M. gave me a prescription for ammonium mandalate, which really didn't help me at all, and if anything it made me feel worse, and I was only taking one 2 or 3 times a day.

I guess this is all of my complaints, and I sure would appreciate it if you could let me know about these things when you have a chance. Thanks so much for all your kindnesses, and I want you to know I sincerely appreciate everything you've done for me.

Remember me to everyone.

This letter illustrates the problems which beset the patient, her husband and two young children during the late advanced period of her illness. On discharge from the hospital it was her wish to return home. The letter also shows the need for a patient at home to have a local physician available and to have the cooperation of a homemaker, visiting nurse and a community health counselor, usually professional with social work background or education in psychology. Patients and families should be told about these resource personnel before the crises occur. Names usually can be suggested by the hospital social worker, the nurse or the secretary of the doctor or the clinic.

The best plan, however, is when the social worker from the hospital setting continues meeting the specific needs and providing emotional support to the end. This ensures optimum continuity of care.

For the patient who does not go home for terminal care there are few resources. Chronic and veterans' hospitals usually have long waiting lists and prefer to take a patient with some chance of rehabilitation. There are some sectarian hospitals, usually Roman Catholic, which will take a patient on a financial sliding scale, and even in a few instances free of charge. But here again the wait for a bed may be a long one.

Nursing homes are another possible facility, but they are increasingly expensive (from $65 to $250 per week), and visiting regularly may disrupt the family's life. In addition, the caregivers on the outside are often concerned with the kind of care their loved one is receiving. But most important is the fact that this type of

placement away from home or hospital where the patient was cared
for previously produces added tensions and feelings of guilt within
the family, even when the patient himself may appear satisfied. A
social worker referred by a member of the hospital team can be of
inestimable value for the patient and the soon-to-be bereaved.

For the patient who remains in the hospital until death, former
caregivers should be alerted. Attending nurses, the social worker
and the most involved family member can interpret the sick
person's need for visits from specific staff members, family and
friends. They also can judge whether visits should be brief or long.
And at this time family members can be helped by attention from
professional or nonprofessional personnel.

As I have said, the patient is totally dependent on his doctor,
nurse and the rest of the medical team when in the hospital, and on
his primary family caregiver and visiting medical personnel when at
home. Occasionally, transfer of the patient to a chronic hospital or
nursing home may be indicated, but usually this is resisted by both
the patient and his family.* I have observed through the years that
the majority of terminal cancer patients wish to remain in their own
homes until the actual dying sets in when they would prefer to be
taken care of in the facility in which they had been treated medically. Families too share this plan if and when it is possible. The patient wants to remain in his familiar setting as long as possible, and
the family strongly wishes to fulfill what they see as their obligation
to take care of him themselves as much as possible. However, the
following two cases demonstrate that each patient's circumstances
require individual evaluation.

John C. was twenty-eight years old, dying of cancer of the rectum. He
had a great deal of pain, a colostomy requiring almost constant dressing,
and, in addition, a difficult temperament. His wife was about his age;
they had two young children. This situation seemed to call for placing
the patient in a chronic hospital. However, his wife, who was well aware
of the prognosis and who would bear the entire burden of his care at
home, refused to place him. They were devoted to one another and to
their children; she was willing to accept the physical and emotional
strain of his care until he died. Wisely, the patient's physician did not
insist on placement but arranged for financial help through the hospital
social work service. He also obtained the services of a visiting nurse and

*R. D. Abrams, G. Jameson, H. Poelman, and S. Snyder. Terminal care: study of 200
patients attending Boston clinics. *N Engl J Med, 232*:719-724, June 21, 1945.

homemaker and arranged counseling so that the couple could meet this crisis in the way they saw best.

The other case, that of Alfred C., illustrates circumstances very different from those in the first case.

> This patient was suffering from inoperable cancer of the jaw, which caused him a great deal of pain. A nerve resection was done, following which he was sent home to live with his wife and two working sons. His wife constantly came to my office in the tumor clinic, complaining of the "excessive" amount of pain her husband was suffering and begging me to place him in a terminal care hospital. It soon became clear that this wife was rejecting her husband so completely that she not only exaggerated his symptoms, but also made him so aware of her disgust that he was willing to be placed, just to get out of a miserable family situation. Happily, this sort of situation is extremely rare.

These two cases demonstrate how easy it is to be mistaken by appearances and how important it is to know each patient as an individual requiring special care to meet his special needs.

## The Patient's Coping Pattern: Silence and Withdrawal

Hackett and Weisman state: "When this illness is fatal, the patient's alienation often mounts to profound loneliness — a state irreversible to drugs."* As I have indicated earlier, the patient withdraws almost totally at this time, but this should not deter his loved ones and friends, or members of the medical team, from expressions of love, sympathy and sorrow. John Hinton, an English psychiatrist, said: "If, together with adequate physical care, the dying person had sufficient human companionship, most of his anguish would be prevented."†

This brings to mind the tragic story of a business executive who knew the truth of his fatal illness. Unfortunately, regarding him as a sensible man, his physician told him he had only two weeks to live. The patient became extremely agitated, so much so that it was deemed necessary to have him speak to another doctor attending him who was willing to set no time limit and to give him

---

*T. P. Hackett, and A. D. Weisman, Treatment of dying. *Curr Psychiatr Ther, 2*:121-126, 1962.

†J. M. Hinton, The physical and mental distress of the dying. *Q J Med, 32*(126):1-21, 1963.

a ray of hope that his life might be extended somewhat. A letter from his wife when he returned home indicated that neither the second physician's comforting words nor the medication was helping as much as anticipated. His wife's exact words, which indicated some reproach, were as follows: "Since we're home Donald has suffered just as he did in the hospital that day he was so bluntly told the whole truth. He is taking Demerol at an alarming rate, I only hope that we can keep him at home, for it's much better for his spirits, I suppose."

Respecting the patient's wish not to talk of his illness does not mean that significant caregivers, now narrowed down to only the most close and necessary, should not be available to visit regularly. It helps the sick person if the others share with him sorrow that medical science has not been able to contend with the progression of his illness. Even visits during which nothing at all may be said show friends' concern and love for the patient, and these are what he needs most. Implied are the words, "What can I do to comfort you?" Thus the family, special friends and members of the medical team reassure the patient that, no matter how he looks or acts, or even if he turns away completely, they will not abandon him; they will continue to care and try to understand. Jean Fox, telling of her nursing experiences, puts it this way:*

> You learn to look beyond the ulcerating foul-smelling breast, beyond the vomiting, the diarrhea, the bladder that goes into spasm, the cough that becomes a paroxysm, the dyspnea that makes the patient gasp for breath.
>
> First, find the person. Reach out with simplicity. Offer the hand, make the gesture that says: I will care, no matter how physically repulsive you become. I will care, no matter how angry, hostile, or depressed you may be. I will care, even though I may not always understand completely.

During these visits, little or nothing may be said. Just the presence of someone caring shows the sick person that those around him continue to love and care for him and to mourn his condition.

I remember the 52-year-old woman who was dying of cancer in

---

*Jean E. Fox, Reflections on cancer nursing. *Am J Nurs,* June 1966.

the hospital. She had been a leader in her society and community affairs, always cheerful and talkative during her earlier hospital admissions. But now, in the final three weeks of her life, she became mute. I visited her every day, sat by her bed holding her hand, and talked to her a little. She seldom replied to anything I said. But, as I left each day, she would express the hope that I would return on the morrow, an indication that these visits were helpful. The hospital staff also appreciated the comfort I was able to give her.

As this example illustrates, the assurance that a caregiver will make another visit to the patient at a specified time in the future, with its implication that the patient will still be alive, is very important. No caregiver should leave a patient's side without telling him exactly when he will return. If he cannot return at all, he should explain and arrange for a replacement before his final visit.

## Does the Dying Patient Want To Communicate with Others about His Illness?

In my study of the cancer patient at the terminal stage I have found that whether he has or has not discussed his fears about death and dying makes no difference in his behavior or ability to accept death. There has been considerable controversy on this point, but I am convinced that the patient who is awake and aware at the time of dying should be permitted by his physician, chaplain, paramedical personnel, friends and family to control his dying himself — to speak of it or not, as he wishes, without prompting. In other words, his caregivers must realize that perhaps it is they who want to talk of death, even though the patient wishes to maintain silence.

If the primary family caregiver in particular has need for greater communication than the patient is willing to permit, a professional caregiver should be available. I have emphasized throughout this book the importance of the chaplain, nurse or social worker to whom the caregiver can turn to talk out his feelings about the patient and find the comfort the patient can no longer give.

Mrs. S. was referred to me by her internist when her feelings of almost complete rejection by her terminally ill husband were more than she could bear. Her husband, an accountant of fifty-six, had not talked with her about his deteriorating illness, his business or his own devotion to her for the past several weeks. She could not take this reversal of confidence by one who had always confided in her. He had been so sensitive to her wishes that he had even arranged a program that allowed her to pick up her earlier musical training. Her whole manner was that of a woman struck not only by the thoughts of inadequacy and impending loss, but also by feelings of exclusion.

My responsibility was to help her to understand her husband's unusual denial (or seeming insensibility to her feelings) and his need to continue to be protected and to protect her from the truth. At first she would not accept the fact that like others with advanced cancer he knew his diagnosis and prognosis, but soon she realized by his anger when she asked him how he felt or how much he weighed (he weighed himself daily) that she was increasing his anxiety and adding to his burden.

I saw Mrs. S. weekly until and after her husband's death (a total of 18 months). We talked especially about what she could anticipate about his reactions as well as her own and what to do about specific problems. Through this communication she became the confident and wise caregiver whom her husband desperately needed. Her husband asked to see me only once just two days before his death. I saw him at his home where he thanked me and inferred that he hoped I would continue to see his wife "later on."

Certainly, the rare patient who indicates a desire to talk of these matters or others concerning his worsening condition should be given the opportunity to do so. He may hint that he wants to talk to a particular person.

An example of a dying patient's need to talk to a specific person was a 50-year-old secretary who said that she suspected and wanted to confirm the truth of her condition, but did not want to disturb the "nice young doctors" who were treating her. With some urging, she did admit that there was one doctor to whom she wanted to talk. He was not her doctor, but she had seen him in the ward and something about him had invited her confidence. I was able to arrange for this doctor, an understanding and warm man, to talk with her. The patient later told me of his visit. There was no need for her to give details, for I saw that her need to discuss her illness had been fulfilled. The subject was never mentioned again.

## Responsibility of Others To Communicate

At times, the caregiver must take some risk for transmitting some of the truth along with support. Recently, more and more of us who care for the dying patient for long or short periods are questioning whether we can continue as in the past to leave all communication about the diagnosis and prognosis to the doctor, the family or the clergy. Nurses, especially, who care for the patient for eight hours or more a day are questioning their responsibility to tell some of the truth to the patient who asks for more information.

In my own experience I felt it only right to say to one patient who asked me why she was not making more progress in spite of following through with all the recommended X-ray treatments and chemotherapeutic drugs, that "we all were very sorry and disappointed that the treatment had not done as much good as we had hoped." She thanked me and died peacefully, without additional sedation, a few days later.

It appears to me that there are times when a patient cannot wait for the "appropriate" informer, but wants to take the opportunity to share her anxieties with whom she chooses at the time she wishes to do so. We must be prepared for these emergencies and have some faith in our ability to meet the crisis.

Thus, we see the patient accepting all kinds of passive, nonverbal help, grateful for what is offered by the doctor, nurse and close family and friends. He continues to regard his doctor as his main source of strength and looks forward to his regular visits.

A surgeon wrote me as follows a few days after we had discussed this need of the terminal patient to have his doctor visit him regularly until the end.

> I recently had the concept of abandonment brought to my attention by a patient, who asked why I had not been by to see him in the previous twenty-four hours. He was in the last week of illness of a rapidly spreading cancer of the pancreas, which I had explored. Prior to that time he had been anxious and hopeful about the possibility of life being prolonged by radiation and chemotherapy.

When that hope was fading, dependency became stronger as evidenced by the worried question about my concern and interest, in spite of the almost daily visits of other consulting physicians. I was the one who knew because I had operated, and if I did not follow the case closely, all hope must be gone. This is a burden, and as you stated, one does find excuses to avoid an unpleasant experience. However, it is with clarification of the needs of the patient, which you so succinctly outlined, that our responsibility is spelled out.

The social worker now is working mainly with the family, although, if she has been a counselor to the patient in the past, she will usually continue her visits. While relying totally now on being cared for, the patient, if he is clearheaded, nevertheless continues to indicate his wishes concerning how, where and by whom he wishes to be cared for. Many of these patients die peacefully, even serenely, if they are allowed to be in control of their own situation and if they can make choices based on their own needs and wishes rather than those of their caregivers.

The reality of the dying cancer patient's situation is just as apparent to him as to others.* I see no reason to interrupt the pattern of withdrawal from that reality unless he himself becomes agitated. In such rare instances the physician in charge may seek consultation from a psychiatrist who is well versed in pharmacological therapy. The important point is that if the patient does not have continuing support from his doctor, direct psychotherapy by a psychiatrist or even spiritual counseling will be of little benefit.

It has been my experience and that of others† that many patients do not reveal that they are having regular visits from the clergy. Is it because their relationship involves confidences never to be shared with others? Perhaps they believe that their expressions of fear of dying, of death and of the hereafter can only be shared with and appreciated by a member of the cloth. Or is it possible that the dying patient feels that if his doctor knows of the clergyman's visits, he may abdicate some of his responsibilities and visit less and less often?

### The Caregivers' Response to the Patient

Whereas formerly in the early advanced stage the patient was

---

*D. Oken, What to tell cancer patients: study of medical attitudes. *JAMA, 175*:1120-1128, 1961.

†L. Feigenberg, Humane Death, Death in Medical Care, Third International Conference on Social Science and Medicine, Elsinore, Denmark, August, 1972.

compulsively active and determined to do everything possible independently, now, as I have stated, he is grateful for the help and support of others and above all the doctor. I have stressed the overriding need for the doctor. This occasionally extends to the nurse, as well.

I have observed that, at the time of dying, the patient seems to regard the doctor as a father figure, and the nurse as a mother figure. I remember the wife of a prominent lawyer who complained to me as her husband lay dying of cancer that his need was not for her, as it had been for almost fifty years, but for the nurse recently assigned to this patient. Perhaps he did not want to reveal himself to his wife at this time, but probably he also did need a maternal figure to help him pass from life to death. When I explained my interpretation to the wife, she was better able to accept the patient's attitude.

The patient wants his family and his familiar home surroundings around him, but he does not want to be involved in any decision making. In fact, the patient begins to separate before final separation and his silence now, as he is dying, is the culmination of this process. A 32-year-old mother of two children, who during two years of illness had repeatedly expressed her realistic concerns regarding her children, stopped talking of them entirely when the late terminal stage was reached. A prominent psychologist turned his face to the wall when visitors came, and another patient, a 40-year-old chemist, pulled the sheet over his face when his wife visited him. This seeming rejection is difficult for the family and friends of the patient; yet, if it is understood as the end product of the long ordeal of illness and suffering, it can be accepted for what it is and not misinterpreted.

## Guidelines for Caregivers

A fundamental concern of all who are involved with the care of a terminal cancer patient is loneliness. The patient, knowing that he is dying, has begun to separate in spirit from those who will survive him, as I have shown. In addition, he suffers from an intense fear of abandonment. He avoids discussing the dismaying aspects of his illness that might trigger emotional crises for himself and his caregivers and thereby increases his sense of aloneness.

These attitudes of course affect the caregivers. Guilt and fear tinge their responses to the patient, changing familiar relationships, injecting uncertainty and uneasiness. Each member of the medical team as well as the family sees the crisis in personal terms and feels alone with his difficulties in coping. This perpetuates the unspoken sense of alienation that is seen so often in cases of terminal cancer.

Counseling help for the family should be available at this time, whether or not they choose to accept it. Whether the patient is being cared for in a nursing facility, chronic hospital or at home, someone — doctor, nurse, social worker, chaplain — should be designated as available to listen to and advise family members. This should not be temporary, "hit-or-miss" assistance, but a well-thought-out, planned support offering specific services that may even be carried over into the period following the patient's death.

When the caregivers know to whom they can turn and what services they can rightfully expect, usually they can carry on without a great deal of outside help. The doctor usually is unable to provide this type of support personally because his time is limited, but he is aware of the capability of other members of the medical team to help. Many people are reluctant to bother the doctor, in any case. Even the president of the board of trustees of a teaching hospital felt this restraint. His wife had acute leukemia, but although he had ready access to all her doctors, he felt compelled to call me each day as one of the medical team to give me the latest findings of her blood condition. He was hopeful when the white cell count was down and hopeless when it was elevated. He knew the implications of his wife's condition, but needed to express himself to someone other than a doctor, someone who would not be "bothered," or perhaps meet his own alternating mood.

All caregivers can best support the patient and help him at this time if they bear in mind the following guidelines.

1. Be available when needed. In particular, try to visit the patient regularly.

2. Accept the patient as he conducts himself: his silence and

withdrawal, his resignation and dependence, his manner and place and time of dying.

3. Take the role the patient assigns you; do not expect too much from the patient or attempt to influence his emotional, social or spiritual outlook. Make it easy for him to accept or reject help.

4. Make sure that the needs of the patient and his family are available when called for, including advance preparation for the death. Be aware of where it may occur, whom to call, funeral arrangements.

5. Remember that everything said and done at this time should be appropriate to the real gravity of the situation. The atmosphere should be such that the patient and his family can grieve together and separately. It is appropriate also for caregivers, both professional and nonprofessional, to show sorrow.

## When Should the Patient Die?

In cancer, death occurs because extensive involvement of the body with disease places too great a strain upon the heart or respiratory system. Just before this happens, the patient most commonly has lapsed into a coma. It is at this time that the question often is raised of keeping the patient alive medically as opposed to allowing him to die in due natural course.

When the patient is obviously failing, perhaps having a great deal of pain or has lapsed into final unconsciousness, the subject of the prolongation of life is generated. This is a highly controversial point. When it is no longer possible to communicate with the patient, then the physician's professional judgment and his knowledge of the family's wishes will guide him in making the decision. Perhaps others on the medical team may not agree with the doctor's choice, but, if he can explain it to them, they at least will be able to understand his reasoning and know that his decision is based on his knowledge and judgment as a physician and on the circumstances of the individual case.

I remember a surgeon who was letting his patient slip away, no longer using any artificial means to prolong life. Her husband knew of the doctor's plan and agreed with it, but the nurses were bewildered that nothing more was being done to keep her alive, and some even appeared angry and unwilling to cooperate. Later, it occurred to me that perhaps some of these misunderstandings could have been avoided if the doctor had simply let his reasons be known to the other members of the medical team, especially the nurses  who are most constantly in attendance on a dying patient and therefore deeply involved in his care and fate.

Another aspect of this decision-making regarding life-prolonging measures at the time of the patient's dying involves whether the family should ever be left with the burden of determining the timing of the patient's death. When this is explained as the final prerogative of the doctor, the family is not burdened with the immediate responsibility of making this crucial decision, nor are they left with a possibly disturbing legacy of doubt regarding the wisdom of their decision in such a situation.

An experience of mine illustrates the soundness and kindness of this approach to this difficult situation. Many years ago I counseled the widowed mother of a 19-year-old boy who had been ill for three years with leukemia and who was dying. This woman had been asked by the resident for help in deciding whether further transfusions of blood should be administered as a means of prolonging her son's life for a period that could range from a few hours to a week.

Because of my long and close relationship with this woman, she was able to ask me, "How can I, his mother, make this choice? How can I live with myself if this decision is left to me?" She intimated, however, that she felt that her son had suffered enough. I telephoned the chief of service and told him of this mother's dilemma. His answer was that he would take care of the situation before the day was out; in his opinion, a mother should not be asked to make this decision. Later, I read on the patient's medical chart this physician's personal order that transfusions be discontinued.

Thus, even in this final decision, the first consideration of the doctor and the patient's family should be the patient's wishes, if he has expressed them at any time during the advancing stage. Too often, the patient's expressed wishes concerning his own death have been "lost in the shuffle."

Recently, Dr. Caroline, a resident at a teaching hospital, has published a tragic experience with such a patient, an old man who had made her promise before his final episode of illness that she would not institute heroic efforts to prolong his life when he was dying. But, when the time came, hospital policy forced her into the decision to make every effort to keep him alive. Many instruments and intravenous appliances were attached to his body, and he was wheeled into another room. Minutes later, when she entered the patient's room, she found him dead. He had pulled out all the needles. On the bedside table she found a note, scrawled in his uneven hand, "Death is not the enemy, Doctor; inhumanity is."*

## After the Death

When a patient is dying of cancer, his family customarily make the necessary arrangements for his funeral in advance, most often according to his stated or implied wishes. When his death takes place, there is little confusion. The appropriate persons are contacted and procedures carried out.

Now the close family draws together for comfort and support. This is a very important phase of recovery from loss. It is remarkable how much strength family members derive from one another and from their memories. Over time these usually concentrate on the happy, fulfilling episodes of the dead person's life with them. That this should be so has been the conscious or unconscious concern of the patient in his preoccupation with his self-image. It is thus that he hopes to live on in their thoughts and affections.

The following letter is a message from a colleague who, after having suffered long years from carcinoma of the breast, wrote it to her friends to be read at her memorial service. I believe it is a fitting conclusion to my book.

> Since no funeral is complete without some words about the departed, I feel it is not out of character to leave a personal message with you, my dear friends. Let this not be a day of sorrow but of thankfulness for a long life, devoted family and friends, a husband

*Nancy S. Caroline, Dying in academe. *The New Physician* (November, 1972), T.N.P.'s Grant Award Winner.

who has loved and enjoyed me for twenty-six years, and for my beloved sons to whom I now wish Godspeed wherever their lives shall take them.

Farewell. No one can perceive the hereafter, but at least I believe firmly that "by their works ye shall know them," and all of us live on through the vessels we have created, the influences we have wrought, the lives we have touched. By this *credo* death is not an end but a way station in the continuum of life, and tragic only if it cuts down a life unfulfilled. So join with me in my serenity, which it will be, when the pain is over. Mourn me briefly, then get on with the business of living, and let it be with a smile, the only thing I would wish for.

"God bless."*

---

*Personal communication, 1972.

# BIBLIOGRAPHY

The references marked with an asterisk (*) are suggested readings.

Abrams, R. D.: Social service and cancer: study of 62 gynecologic patients. J Obstet Gynecol, 50:571-577, November, 1945.

— — —: Social casework with cancer patients. Soc Case, 32(10):425-432, December 1951.

— — —: A social worker examines her activity in clinic study. Selected papers and reports presented at the fiftieth anniversary celebration, Social Service Department. Massachusetts General Hospital, Boston, Massachusetts, October 22, 1955.

— — —: The patient with cancer — his changing pattern of communication. N Engl J Med, 274:317-322, February 10, 1966.

—: Denial and depression in the terminal cancer patient — a clue for management. Psychiatr Q, 45:394-404, November 3, 1971.

— — —: The responsibility of social work in terminal cancer. In Psycho-social Aspects of Terminal Care. New York, Columbia University Press, 1971.

— — —, and Dana, B.: Social work in the process of rehabilitation. Soc Work, October 1957.

— — —, and Finesinger, J. E.: Guilt reactions in patients with cancer. Cancer, 6:474-482, May 1953.

— — —, and Hindley, M.: Bereavement in cancer — adjustment processes of surviving spouses under age 45. In press.

— — —, and Hindley, M.: Helps and hindrances in the management of the cancer patient, A guide to total treatment. To be published, 1976.

— — —, Jameson, G., Poelman, H., and Snyder, S.: Terminal care: study of 200 patients attending Boston clinics. N Engl J Med, 232:719-724, June 21, 1945.

Adair, F. E.: Cancer in our breast: interview with John Gunther. Women's Home Companion, February 1954.

Barckley, V.: What can I say to the cancer patient? J Pract Nurs, April 1964.

— — —: The crises in cancer. Am J Nurs, February 1967

Cassem, N. H.: New hospital practices reflect a need to help dying patients prepare for death. The New York Times, January 21, 1973.

Chicago Tumor Institute Report, 1963. Unpublished.

Conjugal Bereavement Study, Laboratory of Community Psychiatry, Harvard Medical School, Boston, Massachusetts. New Series, 1968.

*Fairbanks, R. J.: Administering to the sick. The Starr Lecture, Trinity College, Toronto, Canada, September 1947.

Feigenberg, Loma: Humane Death. Death in Medical Care, International Conference on Social Science and Medicine, Elsinore, Denmark, August 1972

Finesinger, J. E.: Medical history taking, San Fransisco, California, September 1949, unpublished.

— — —, Shands, H. C., and Abrams, R. D.: Managing the emotional problems of the cancer patient. Clinical Problems in Cancer Research — Sloan-Kettering Seminar, Memorial Hospital, New York, 1951.

Fox, J. E.: Reflections in cancer nursing. Am J Nurs, June 1966.

Glick, I., Weiss, R. and Parkes C. Murray: The First Year of Bereavement. New York, Wiley and Sons, 1974.

Grof, S., Pahnke, W. N., Goodman, L. E., and Kurland, A. A.: LSD — Psychedelic drug-assisted psychotherapy in patients with terminal cancer, Part 2. JAMA, 212:1856, 1970.

Hackett, R. P., and Weisman, A. D.: Psychiatric management of operative syndromes. II. Psychodynamic factors in formulation and management. Psychosom Med, 22:356-372, 1960.

— — —, and Weisman, A. D.: Treatment of dying. Curr Psychiatr Ther, 2:121-126, 1962.

Hinton, J. M.: The physical and mental distress of the dying. Q J Med, 32(126):1-21, 1963.

*Kubler-Ross, E.: On Death and Dying. New York, The Macmillan Company, 1969.

Leigh, Hoyle: Psychiatric liason on a neoplastic inpatient service. Psychiatr in Medicine, Vol. 4, pages 147-154, Spring, 1973.

*Lifton, R. J.: On death and death symbolism: Hiroshima disaster. Psychiatry, 27:191-210, 1964.

*Mendelsohn, J.: What a piece of work is man. In White, L. P. (Ed.): Care of Patients with Fatal Illness. Ann N Y Acad Sci, New York, 164:818-821, December 19, 1969.

Oken, D.: What to tell cancer patients: Study of medical attitudes. JAMA, 175:1120-1128, 1961.

*Parad, H. J., and Caplan, G.: A framework for studying families in crisis. In Parad, H. J. (Ed.): Crisis Intervention. New York, Family Service Association of America, 1965.

Saunders, C.: The treatment of intractable pain in terminal cancer. Proc R Soc Med, 56(3):195-197, 1963.

— — —: The last stages of life. Am J Nurs, 65:70-75, 1965.

*Schoenberg, B., Carr, A., Peretz, H., and Kutscher, A. H. (Eds.): Psycho-Social Aspects of Terminal Care. New York, Columbia University Press, 1972.

Shands, H., Finesinger, J. E., Cobb, S., and Abrams, R. D.: Psychological mechanisms in patients with cancer. Cancer, 4:1159-1170, 1951.

*Wahl, C. W.: The physician's treatment of the dying patient. In White, L. P. (Ed.): Care of Patients with Fatal Illness. Ann N Y Acad Sci, 164:759-772, December 19, 1969.

Weisman, A. D.: On Dying and Denying. New York, Behavioral Publications, 1973.

— — —, and Hackett, T. P.: Predilection to death: death and dying as psychiatric problem. Psychosom Med, 23:232-256, 1961.

*WGBH: Nursing Home Reports, Program #11. The terminal cancer patient. Eastern Educational Network (Channel 2), April 1968.

*White, L. P.: The self-image of the physician and the care of dying patients. In Care of Patients with Fatal Illness. Edited by L. P. White. Annals of the New York Academy of Sciences, New York, December 19, 1969, 164:822-837.

*— — — (Ed.): Care of Patients with Fatal Illness. Ann N Y Acad Sci, 164(3):635-896, December 19, 1969.

# SUBJECT INDEX

## A

American Cancer Society, xix, xxv, 20
Ammonium mandalate, 73
Anesthesia
dread of, 6

## B

Biopsy
definition of, 9
Blue Cross and Blue Shield, 18
Bufferin, 33

## C

Cancer
causes of, xv, 17
death and (*see* Life, prolongation of)
diabetes and, comparison between, xv,
31 (*see also* Cancer patient, cured)
diagnosis of, 3 (*see also* Examination,
delay in medical)
reaction to, family, 15
reaction to, patient, 15-16 (*see also*
Hospital release, reaction to, patient)
significance of, 4
testing, for, 9
disclosure of, physician, 3, 10-11, 16
reaction to, patient, xiii-xiv, xvi
dread of, xv
factors involving, hereditary
discussion of, 17
heart disease and, comparison between, xv, 31
incidence of, xi, xv
metastasization of, 29
phases of, emotional, 5
stage of, advanced (*see also* Cancer
patient, advanced)
characteristics of, 62-65

definition of, 41
description of, xix
disclosure of, physician, 45-47
expectancy, determination of life,
41
periods of, 42
phases of, discussion of, 59
reactions during, caregivers, 42 (*see
also* Caregiver)
reactions during, family, 41-42,
51-52 (*see also* Family)
reactions to, patient, 50-51
rejection during, significance of, 41
treatment, rationale for, 41, 47
stage of, late advanced (*see also* Cancer
patient, late advanced)
characteristics of, 70
definition of, 70
reactions to, family, 70
treatment, discussion of, 71
stage of, localized (*see also* Cancer
patient)
description of, xix
treatment of, 9
treatment of, follow-up, 37
stage of, regional involvement, 25 (*see
also* Cancer patient)
definition of, 29
description of, xix
disclosure of, physician, 30
reactions to, family, 30
reactions to, patient, 30-34, 38-39
reactions to, physician, 30-31 (*see
also* Cancer patient, relationship
between physician and)
treatment, methods of, 30
stages of, xvii, xix
symptoms of, 7
discovery of, 4 (*see also* Cancer,
disclosure of)
symptoms of, reporting of
attitude toward, physician, 8-9

treatment of
  avoidance of, patient, 16-17
  diet and, 33-34
  disclosure of, physician, 19
  effects of, side, 9, 30
  faith in, patient, 19
  fear of, patient, 17
  involvement in, patient, xi
  reaction to, patient, 18-19
Cancer, breast (*see also* Mastectomies)
  diagnosis of
  reaction to, patient, 16
  life expectancy
  discussion of, xvi
Cancer, lung (*see also* Cancer, diagnosis
    of)
  life expectancy
  discussion of, xvi
Cancer, ovarian, 33
Cancer, skin
  cure, rate of, xv
Cancer patient
  caregivers and, relationship between
    factors affecting, 37 (*see also* Care-
      giver, the)
  chaplain and, relationship between,
    14-15 (*see also* Chaplain, the)
  death of
  reactions to, family (*see* Death)
  dignity, maintenance of
    important of, viii
  family and, relationship between, 38
    (*see also* Family)
  nurse and, relationship between, 12-13
    (*see also* Nurse)
  physician and, relationship between,
    ix, xvii-xviii, 19, 33
    factors affecting, 31, 34-35, 36, 38
    importance of, 35, 43-44
  problems of, financial, 18, 59-60
  reaction to, caregiver, 17-18
  reaction to, family, xxi-xxii, 17-18
  reactions of, emotional, viii
  readjustment of, 20
  social worker and, relationship be-
    tween, 13-14, 80 (*see also* Social
    worker)
  treatment of, follow-up, 21 (*see also*
    Cancer, treatment of)

Cancer patient, advanced
  chaplain and, relationship between, 58
    (*see also* Chaplain)
  counselor and, relationship between,
    57-58
  dignity, maintenance of
    importance of, 42
  family of
    counselor and, relationship between,
      57-58
    disclosure to, 52-53
    physician and, relationship between,
      51-52
  life-style of
    changes, discussion of, 59
  physician and, relationship between,
    48-50, 66
    factors affecting, 44-45
  problems, emotional
    discussion of, 48-49
  reactions of, emotional, xx, 60-66
  reactions to, caregiver, 54-55, 61 (*see
    also* Caregiver)
  reactions to, family, 54-55
  suicide and, discussion of, 65-66
  treatment of
    choice of, factors affecting, 47 (*see
      also* Treatment)
    types, discussion of, 47-48
Cancer patients, cured
  reactions of, psychological, 21-22
  reactions to, co-worker, 23
  readjustments of, career, 22
  readjustments of, physical, 22
Cancer patients, late advanced
  care of, home
    planning of, 72-73, 74-75
  care of, hospital
    discussion of, 73-74
  care of, nursing home
    discussion of, 73-74
  caregiver and, relationship between, 79
  family and, relationship between
    importance of, 76
  fear, discussion of, 81-82
  nurse and, relationship between, 79-81
  physician and, relationship between,
    79-81
  reactions to, caregiver, 77-79

# AUTHOR INDEX

# ABOUT THE AUTHOR

Ruth D. Abrams has been a pioneer in the counseling of cancer patients and their families since June, 1945 when she had her first article published in *The New England Journal of Medicine.* During World War II when her doctor-husband, Archie A. Abrams, was in service and her two children were in elementary school, she received her Master's in Social Work from Simmons. She is a charter member of the ACSW (Academy of Certified Social Workers). In 1966, Simmons School of Social Work awarded her the Harriet M. Bartlett Prize for her article, "The Patient with Cancer—His Changing Pattern of Communication," published in *The New England Journal of Medicine* in February, 1966. Actually, this article was the genesis of this, her most recent publication, NOT ALONE WITH CANCER.

Mrs. Abrams was a member of the Social Service Department of the Massachusetts General Hospital where she became clinical supervisor. As a research social worker she worked jointly on projects related to cancer with the Departments of Psychiatry and Gynecology. From her wide experience came numerous articles which appeared in various journals such as *Social Casework, Cancer, Psychiatric Quarterly,* and *Annals of the New York Academy of Science.* She has served on the Advisory Committee of the Social Service Committee of the American Cancer Society, Inc. (National) and more recently on their program committee. In addition, she has lectured and participated in programs throughout this country and abroad, in Scotland, The Netherlands, and England.

At one time Mrs. Abrams was Assistant Professor of Social Work at the Boston University School of Social Work and Research Assistant at the Harvard School of Public Health. Her most recent affiliation was with the Conjugal Bereavement Study, Laboratory of Community Psychiatry at the Harvard Medical School. Presently she is a mental health counselor for the cancer patient and his family, and a lecturer and consultant to the health professions. She continues independent study and writing which focuses on ensuring the comfort and self-respect of the patient and of all those concerned with his care.

In 1975 Mrs. Abrams was a Site Visitor for the National Cancer Institute, U.S. Department of Health, Education and Welfare. In that same year she became the first recipient of the Distinguished Service Award granted by The Foundation of Thanatology, New York. In recognition of this award, a colleague, Elizabeth R. Prichard, Director of Social Service at Presbyterian Hospital, New York, wrote the following letter to Mrs. Abrams:

> It was a proud time for all of us to have a social worker receive the first award of the Foundation of Thanatology. The Social Work Symposium was in a sense a culmination of the work in which you were a pioneer. For it was you who alone for many years laid the foundation on which our efforts can now be built. We are indebted to you for identifying the in-depth areas of concern to patients and their families and formulating techniques for case work treatment, and demonstrating the social work contribution. We can all admire your vision and courage in following through what until now was an unpopular field of inquiry. It is a form of professional discipline which is more often talked about, but little results are seen. I have been particularly impressed by your ability to combine professional skill with a profound sense of caring. This is really the core of concern and why many social workers were fearful of working with the terminal patient. You have shown us the way, we are now more comfortable and thus eternally grateful to you. And when you received the award, it was at that moment that a milestone had been reached for all of us, and the profession of Social Work.

# NOT ALONE WITH CANCER

"Cancer is a fearful word for a patient and his family, and often also for the professional care-giver — the nurse, social worker and physician. For even those trained in the care of the living have been taught little about the care of the dying. This paperback is of convenient pocket size, less than 100 pages, with a commendably selected bibliography. In the preface, Mrs. Abrams, a professional psychiatric social worker, explains that it grew out of her 25 years' experience dealing with patients with cancer and their families. It is intended as a thoughtful and practical guide to help break down the wall of silence and despair that too long has been the burden of the patient with cancer and those who care for him. There is a message here for all those involved in care-giving — above all, that the patient should be allowed to choose his own way of coping, when he knows what he is facing — whether with silence and withdrawal, denial or a seeming rejection of those he has loved. But this is not a book about an incurable situation — far from it. The first chapter deals with a curable neoplasm, the first stage, when the growth is localized. It describes what most patients fear, how they express it, and in what way the family or the doctor may find an answer.

"The second chapter treats the stage of regional involvement — when it is apparent that the tumor has extended beyond its original location. The outlook is no longer good; yet therapy carries the hope of partial if not total success. It may be necessary to call in new specialists, a threat to the delicacy of the initial doctor-patient relation. If dependence on the physician who offers that hope is important in this stage of the disease, it is absolutely mandatory in the advanced stages of cancer.

"The last two chapters, taking up 40 pages of text, are devoted to the time when there is no way to stop further spread of the disease. Mrs. Abrams divides this into the time of telling and waiting, and finally, the time of dying. How does the family deal with the patient's feeling of rejection, usually present, whether or not it is openly expressed? And how much of the truth must the doctor tell his patient? What is the role of principal family care-giver, the social worker, the nurse, the clergy? Finally, in a description of the effort by all those who care, to allow the patient to live his remaining days with as much dignity and satisfaction as possible, the author draws from her own deep and rich experience. 'By spelling out what happens at the end of life,' says Robert S. Weiss in the Foreword, 'Mrs. Abrams forces us to recognize that time has us, too, in its grip, and that we, too, will have our confrontation with death.' This is a book that we all have wanted for a long time. It is a precious guide for everyone — a positive assurance that no one need feel left alone to face a cancer."

Somers H. Sturgis, M.D.
Professor of Gynecology (Emeritus)
Harvard Medical School
*The New England Journal of Medicine*
Vol. 292, No. 23 (June 5, 1975)

**CHARLES C THOMAS • PUBLISHER • SPRINGFIELD • ILLINOIS**